The 30-Day Whole Food Challenge:

A Guide to a "Whole" New You!

Table of Contents

Introduction i
Chapter 1: What Is the Whole Food Challenge? 1
Chapter 2: Benefits of the Whole Food Challenge 8
Chapter 3: Food Items to Avoid and Why 15
Chapter 4: Persistence Is the Key to Resistance 23
Chapter 5: Foods You Can Enjoy 29
Chapter 6: The 30-Day Challenge 35
Chapter 7: Kitchen Essentials 18
Chapter 8: Whole Food Recipes for a "Whole" New You 21
Conclusion 174

© Copyright 2018 by _____
- All rights reserved.

The following eBook is reproduced with the goal of providing information that is as accurate and reliable as possible. Regardless, purchasing this eBook can be seen as consent to the fact that both the publisher and the author of this book are in no way experts on the topics discussed within and that any recommendations or suggestions that are made herein are for entertainment purposes only. Professionals should be consulted as needed prior to undertaking any of the action endorsed herein.

This declaration is deemed fair and valid by both the American Bar Association and the Committee of Publishers Association and is legally binding throughout the United States.

Furthermore, the transmission, duplication or reproduction of any of the following work including specific information will be considered an illegal act irrespective of if it is done electronically or in print. This extends to creating a secondary or tertiary copy of the work or a recorded copy and is only allowed with an expressed written consent from the Publisher. All additional right reserved.

The information in the following pages is broadly considered to be a truthful and accurate account of facts ,and as such any inattention, use or misuse of the information in question by the reader will render any resulting actions solely under their purview. There are no scenarios in which the publisher or the original author of this work can be in any fashion deemed liable for any hardship or damages that may befall them after undertaking information described herein.

Additionally, the information in the following pages is intended only for informational purposes and should thus be thought of as universal. As befitting its nature, it is presented without assurance regarding its prolonged validity or interim quality. Trademarks that are mentioned are done without written consent and can in no way be considered an endorsement from the trademark holder.

Introduction

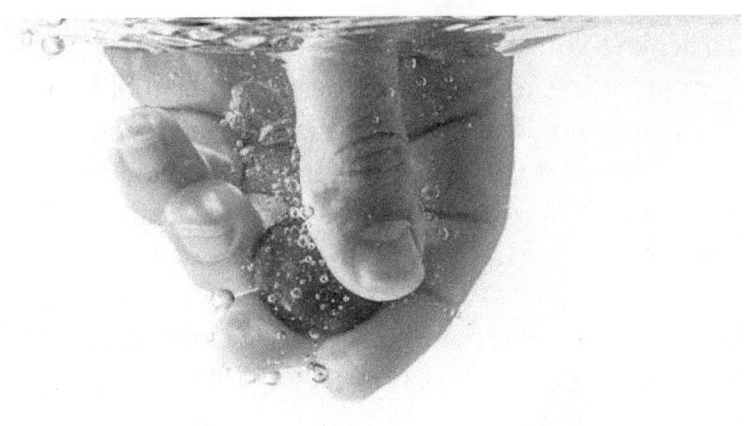

Congratulations on downloading *The 30-Day Whole Food Challenge: A Guide to a "Whole" New You*, and thank you for doing so.

The following chapters will teach you how to lose weight and become healthier using the 30-day whole food diet .If you want to lose weight but you're unsure what to eat to stay healthy and achieve results—or if you have started a diet but are having a hard time sticking to the meal plan—this book will help you solve those problems.

Before you begin any diet, it's important to understand that for it to be successful, you must have the right mindset, information, and understanding. A good place to start would be to learn what kind of food to eat and how to eat them.

To achieve your desired weight, a foundation of healthy eating, and that includes knowing about how much you should eat (portion size). When it comes to everything that you eat, whether it's a meal or a snack, it's crucial that you learn how to plan for health and not convenience.

If you have tried other diets before, you might be aware of one common factor they share—that is, they don't necessarily teach you about how to pay equal attention to the effects on the mind and the body during the process. It definitely takes discipline to eat healthy to stay healthy, but it doesn't have to be stressful.

Leading industry experts believe that when we consume whole foods, we give our bodies the best defense for fighting off diseases and that it helps with the overall improvement of our health. With this 30-day whole food challenge guide, you are not only going to learn what to stay away from, you are also going to benefit from the breakfast, lunch, dinner, snack, and dessert recipes within its pages. We have also provided you with tons of information on the 30-day challenge and its key benefits. We are confident that following this guide will lead to a "whole" new and healthier you.

As there are plenty of books on this subject on the market, we thank you again for choosing this one. Every effort was made to ensure it is full of as much useful information as possible. Enjoy!

Chapter 1: What Is the Whole Food Challenge?

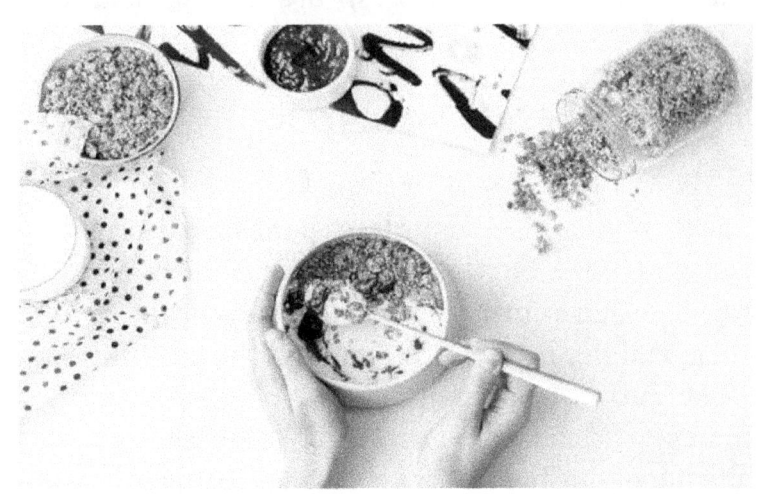

Definition of Whole Food

Whole food, according to extensive research, made its first appearance in *The Farmer*, a magazine published quarterly by F. Newman Turner. Turner was one of the world's first organic farmers who pioneered the "Whole Foods" movement.

In 1946, Turner and his associates defined "whole foods" as

"...mature produce of field, orchard, or garden without subtraction, addition, or alteration grown from seed without chemical dressing, in fertile soil manure solely with animal and vegetable wastes, and composts there from, and ground, raw rock and without chemical manures, sprays, or insecticides."

Whole30®

The aforementioned report was published decades ago, and today, numerous health blogs, diets, and regimens have emerged to change the way we eat, shop, and live healthily. As stated in the introduction, most "fad" diets fall short of combining the correct mindset with action plans. Luckily, Melissa H art wig and her ex-husband decided to take this long-forgotten way of living and eating and created a new way of life called Whole30®.

The relatable story behind the movement began in 2009. Melissa was working full time as an insurance agent in southern New Hampshire and was also heavily involved in learning about living and eating healthy. In her spare time, she was running a consultation practice for fitness education and nutrition.

Melissa first came out with the Whole30® concept on her fitness blog after realizing that many of her readers were suffering from the same things. It was also at that time that her ex-husband, Dallas, was struggling with chronic shoulder pain and began to look at which foods were causing him to have flare-ups (inflammation). The challenge called Whole30® was born mainly to solve these common health concerns.

The pair decided to test out Dallas' research and analysis of food properties and cut out every single food that Dallas had identified as pot entailing inflammation triggers. Afterward, one at a time, he began to eat them again to determine which ones were causing the most issues.

Earlier, we mentioned the mental aspect of dieting. Most of us don't usually take into account that the food we eat can affect not only our physical health but also our mood and behavior .That existence of that connection is exactly what this experiment had approved. Melissa noticed an increase in positive mood swings and a higher energy level after the change in her ex-husband's diet. According to her, the observable effects deeply affected the way she related with food.

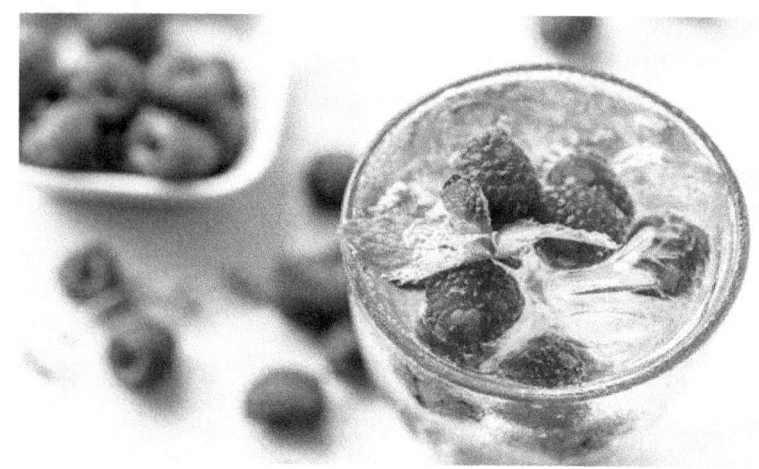

Detoxify and Purify

The main concept of the 30-day whole food diet involves reboot in one's entire lifestyle and eliminating bad eating habits .The process all begins with a thorough full-body detoxification. You should note that regardless of the diet you ultimately decide to commit to, it is of utmost importance that you detoxify your body first.

This particular challenge is different in that it calls for a continuous detoxification, not just the once. Our bodies must not only rid itself of foods that are causing us physical and psychological harm but also keep away from them thereafter. Detoxifying is also extremely important for those suffering from any type of chronic illness or pain.

Detox here means ridding your body of wastes that have built up. There are toxic chemicals in everything we see, touch, and eat on a daily basis, and according to numerous doctors, research studies, and even the FDA, these chemicals are literally attacking our bodies—from our inner organs down to our hair and skin. Autoimmune diseases, food allergies, digestive troubles, dementia—just about every known disease can trace back its root cause to toxins .If that's not enough to make you want to detoxify, then what will?

The Whole Food Challenge Explained

Let's face it, who doesn't like a little sugar with their cereal or an extra block of butter on their dinner rolls? The problem is, these particular types of food groups are the ones that have the biggest impact on your body and energy levels yet many of their effects go unnoticed.

Compared to other diets, the great thing about the whole food challenge is that there are no videos to watch, no books to read, no gadgets to buy, and no supplements to take. The whole food challenge is more than a fad; it is a way of life. Honestly speaking, it all boils down to three simple words: eat better food.

The whole food challenge is all about eating food that are as close to their original, organic state and form as possible instead of eating the processed foods that dominate supermarkets everywhere. Not only is this process designed to help you lose weight, it's also designed to guide you in developing a lifestyle that reduces pain and risk of illness while keeping the weight off.

The reason eating whole foods is good for us is because they have not been "messed with." They don't have added sugar, fat, or salt, and they don't contain preservatives that can ruin a diet. As reported by Dr. Mark Hyman, you don't necessarily need a lot of medicine to treat the common illnesses that people suffer from today, you can combat disease by eating food rich in vitamins, minerals, omega-3 fatty acids, and phytonutrients derived from "phyto"—the Greek word for plant.

Eating processed foods over an extended period not only adds to our weight but also causes hormonal and blood sugar imbalances. These can result in two things:

- An "empty" feeling in your stomach even after you've eaten.
- The release of more feel-good chemicals in your brain that tricks you into thinking you should eat more processed food.

These factors can lead you to eat more and more of the same food that makes you fat. In turn, that can lead to a slight or, in some cases, extreme obesity.

In a recent study, scientists found what is called *glucagon*, a hormone in the body that helps to suppress our appetite and is responsible for making us feel full. This particular hormone is produced in the pancreas. Some studies suggest that an imbalance with this hormone can cause extensive health problems in addition to increased weight.

Ready to throw out those chips yet? No? If you need some more convincing, let's discuss the health benefits of the 30-day whole food challenge a bit more in detail.

Chapter 2: Benefits of the Whole Food Challenge

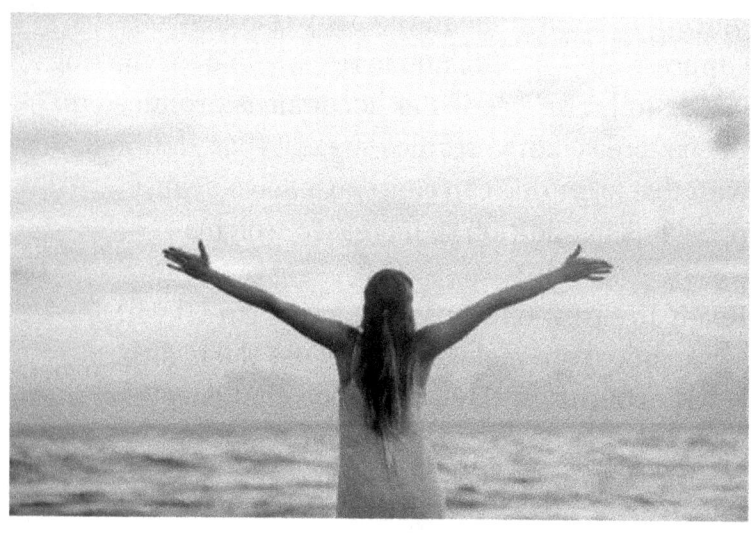

Mental Health Benefits of Eating Whole Foods

Our brain has no "off" switch. Something has to keep you breathing even while you sleep, right? The brain controls our heartbeat, senses, thoughts, and movements every minute, every second of every single day. Yet even though the brain never stops working—not even for a split second—it is often one of the most under-appreciated parts of our body. Much like the workings of a sports car, the brain requires premium fuel to keep running smoothly. Food that are high in fatty acids, such as those loaded with too much sugar or salt, and not in vitamins and minerals, do not provide us with the ample fuel our brain needs to function and perform at its best.

Our sleep cycle and our feelings of hunger are controlled by a neurotransmitter called serotonin. About 95% of this substance is produced in the gastrointestinal tract, which might explain why hunger can affect our emotions .Our digestive system also houses lots of "good" bacteria that are essential to maintaining good health. They act as the army of our stomach lining, protecting our digestive system against the "bad" bacteria trying to get into our bodies. The good bacteria are not only responsible for reducing chronic pain flare-ups, they also partly dictate how quickly you digest and absorb nutrients from food as well as act as the direct highway from your gut to your brain.

There is an increasing number of research studies that show that people who eat healthier are typically 30% less depressed than those who do not. Not only does eating healthy reduce depression, it has also been found to reduce the number of anxiety attacks, hyperactivity (ADD/ADHD), and even bipolar episodes in sufferers. Mood swings, that roller coaster ride of emotions with internal dips and climbs, are associated with unregulated sugar levels in our body. A recent news report on CNN stated that certain foods help boost our brain function and our body remain active.

There are currently over 300 million people in the world suffering from depression, and processed food has been attributed to an increase in teen depression, in particular. If you have teenagers in your household, this is especially important to take note of. What we refer to as the "western diet, "which is typically made up of processed food and food that do not contain quality nutrients and minerals, is a big part of what is causing the imbalance in your mood and even your brain function. You must have heard the saying". You are what you eat" at least once in your life. No truer words have been spoken.

Start keeping a journal of how you feel after eating certain foods and document common patterns. Do not just describe that initial feeling. Dive deeper into your thought patterns and try to notice the times when some of your feelings might be disturbed because of the feeling of hunger or a need for instant gratification. Document how you feel once your body has had the chance to digest and break the food you consumed; pay attention to what happens once the food has gone from your gut to your brain.

When keeping a food journal, remember to write down every single thing you eat. If you can keep a journal in your briefcase or in your purse, take it with you wherever you go so you won't miss recording anything. When you are drained and tired, you will have a tendency to forget. A common thing people do to document their Whole foods challenge is making columns.

Physical Health Benefits of Eating Whole Foods

Now that you understand that what you eat can affect your mood and your behavior, let's talk about how eating the right and wrong types of food can affect your body. When we eat whole foods, we are doing what nature intended: that we eat foods that are as close to their organic state as possible.

The concept behind whole food eating and dieting is the natural balance that keeps our bodies aligned and functioning at maximum capacity and enables us to be more active. Processed foods that have been changed from their original state, i.e., something has been either removed or added, goes against the natural balance. Our bodies are not designed to process these foods well.

The food we eat is not just supposed to curb our hunger, it is meant to nourish the cells that make up the human body, and there is a direct correlation between the food we eat and the "health cells" of each particular food group. For example, if you eat a lot of junk food, packaged food, or sugar/salt-fueled food, the cells in your body are not reproducing at the normal rate required for healthy living. The opposite is true when you eat healthy. Your cells reproduce at normal rates.

The whole food challenge focuses on the prevention, not the cure, because if we prevent these diseases in the first place, no cure will be needed. As a society, we have long veered off the path of organic eating and instead opted for convenience, ease of access, and pleasure. Societies who live away from civilization and still eat whole foods do not have nearly the amount of health problems that those of us in western civilizations do, and they do not suffer from depression nearly as much as well.

"The cure is the same as the prevention. Let food be thy medicine."~Hippocrates

I think we can all agree that when presented with a baked potato or a bag of chips, the better choice would be the baked potato. If you use that same logic when deciding on your food choices, it will definitely benefit you and your overall health in the long run. Read the nutrition label on the package very carefully. Does the list of added ingredients go from top to bottom? How many items have been added or removed to take it away from its original state? If I eat this, will it affect my gut, which has a direct highway to my brain and can thereby affect my mood and behavior? Asking these questions every time you eat will eventually lead to better eating, ultimately affecting your long-term health.

Long-Term Benefits of Eating Whole Food

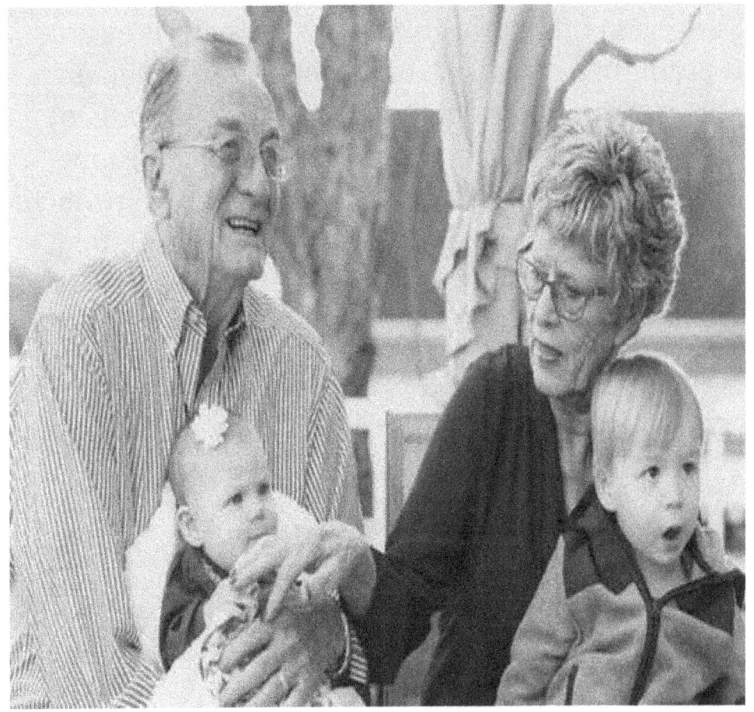

A well-balanced diet is the new fountain of youth. Doctors suggest that, as we get older, 1800 calories per day is the average amount we can take in. What's more important than the number is how we break up those calories for healthier, longer living.

Think about the parts of our bodies that require different kinds of attention as we age. You would want to focus on eating enough protein to enhance your muscles or drink and eat enough calcium to strengthen your bones and maintain a healthy heart. Following these guidelines can also help you control your weight.

Please don't think we are saying that aging is a curse. It is not. In fact, it's one of the most beautiful natural progressions of life. However, it is never too late to start eating and living healthier. Remember, eating whole foods can help you do just that. It has proven to help decrease blood sugar, provide better digestion, give you more energy, relieve you of chronic pain, and give you a full and satisfied feeling.

Chapter 3: Food Items to Avoid and Why

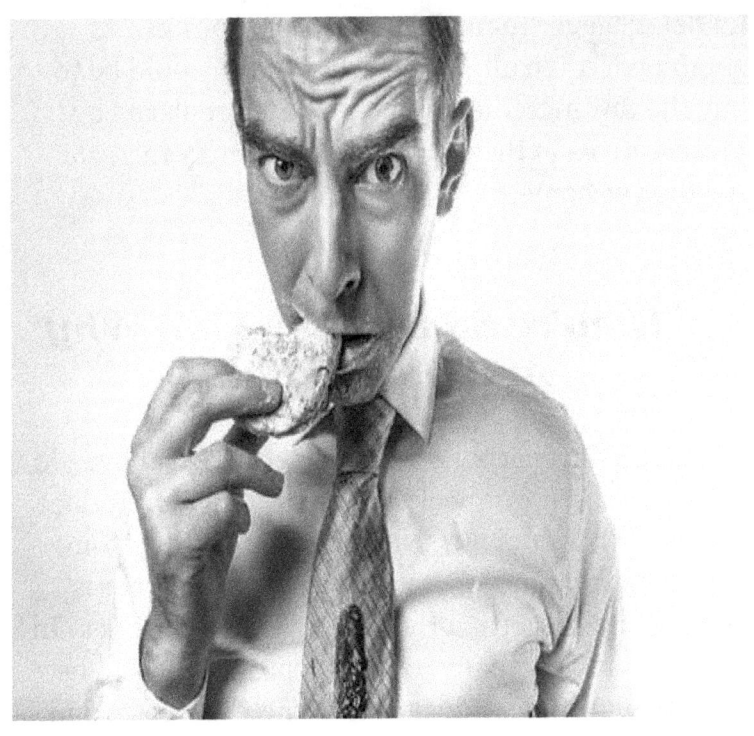

We've already mentioned this multiple times, but the number one type of food you want to avoid are the processed ones. Imagine these being manufactured, reconstructed, and packaged in a factory somewhere and compare that to food being grown from the ground. Food corporations have been known to substitute ingredients to make their products cheaper to manufacture. As mentioned in Chapter 2, it pays to read all the ingredients and information listed on every package. By doing so, you'll find that these are generally not healthy at all. Remember that we need good, cell-rich food and that cheap ingredients simply don't cut it. In the long run, your hospital bill may end up being bigger than all your grocery choices combined. All in all, the smartest move would be to buy the raw ingredients that had been replaced by preservatives in these productsand simply recreate the food at home.

If They're So Bad For You, Why Are They Legal?

Unfortunately, corporations, as mentioned above, do not think about our health when deciding to produce products. They do, however, consider their bottom line. What that means for the average consumer is that we end up getting the shorter end of the stick. In order for any company to make a profit, it has to be able to make the product at extremely low costs and sell it for a higher price. That is exactly why they prefer to take shortcuts on the quality of the ingredients they use. Please don't assume we are lumping all food corporations together as being inconsiderate money-making machines. The good news is that not all companies think nor operate like this, and while they manufacture and distribute their products in similar packaging, they often get sold in places like Whole Foods, GNC, and other health food stores.

However, the selection process is far from simple. As we mentioned earlier, not all products sold in health food stores are what we need for our bodies. Do not let its existence in a healthier location or aisle distract you. Major corporations are famous for buying out smaller health food stores that fail to survive amid stiff competition, and they become huge profit makers. It is ultimately up to each of us to be smart, savvy shoppers.

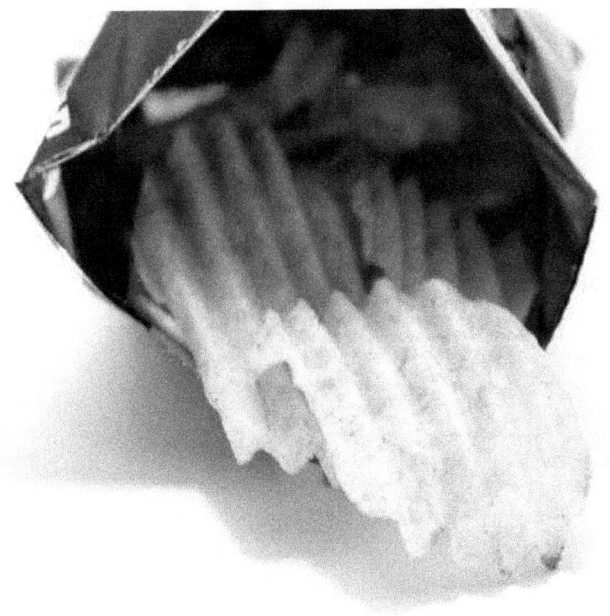

Earlier in this book, we gave you a few questions to ask yourself as you read product labels and practice vigilance about what you and your family members eat. Here are a couple more useful questions that can be useful for determining the quality and the benefits of what you're buying:

- Are all the ingredients listed on the product label organic or non-GMO?

- Could you easily replicate any item in your home?

If you can answer yes to those questions, by all means, purchase that product with peace of mind. It is items such as this that will help the nourishment of your body.

If you cannot answer yes to those questions, on the other hand, consider if this product is going to be healthy for your family and for yourself. The quick answer here is a simple no. We suggest that you choose a healthier alternative. Always keep in mind that your long-term mental and physical health depends on these daily decisions.

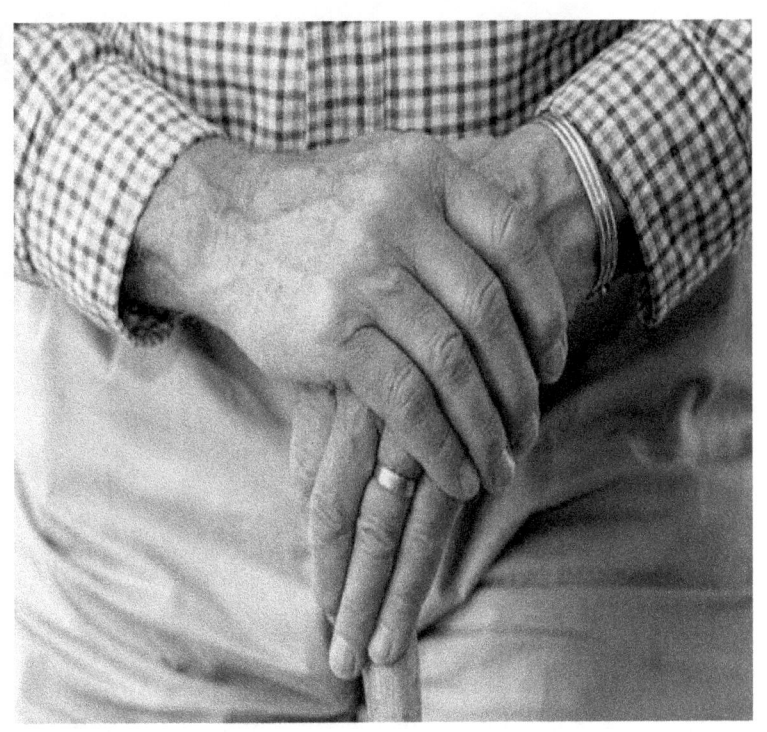

Foods and Ingredients to Avoid

Let's talk about the types of food and ingredients that you will want to stay away from after finding them listed in product labels. Keep in mind that the majority of processed foods are full of additives and fillers.

Fillers: Also known as additives, fillers help to beef up the actual weight of certain foods with cheaper ingredients, and doing so helps cut manufacturing costs for most major companies. An example of a food that uses fillers: most Greek yogurts.

Preservatives: This is one of the scary ones. Preservatives are chemicals meant to preserve the shelf life of the food. Included here are benzoates, which, is another way to refer to sodium or salt, and benzoic acids. Other examples are nitrates, also a form of salt that is commonly known as sodium nitrate, and sulfates also known as sulfur dioxide, which is the least desirable. Yes, these harmful chemicals are in our food—even the ones we give our children—and we often consume them in haste.

Artificial colors and flavors: These are known to cause just about everything from hyperactivity to severe allergic reactions to even the dreaded C word: cancer.

Artificial sweeteners: Ditch your Equal and your Sweet-n-Low immediately. According to an article by Harvard Medical School,

"Frequent use of these hyper-intense sweeteners may limit tolerance for more complex tastes. That means people who routinely use artificial sweeteners may start to find less intensely sweet foods, such as fruit, less appealing and un sweet foods, such as vegetables, downright unpalatable."

What that means is that the more you use these artificial sweeteners, the less likely you will be able to even tolerate the taste of fruits and vegetables. Not a good thing if you want to adopt a whole food lifestyle.

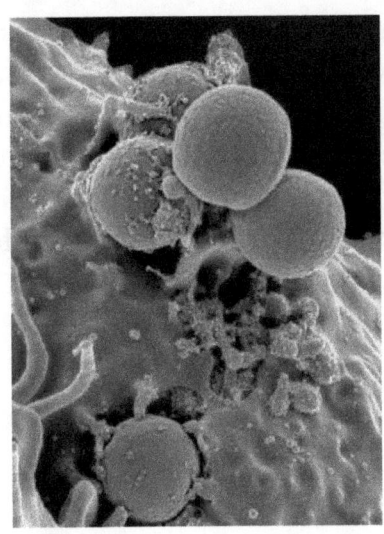

GMOs: This stands for genetically modified organisms. There are tons of arguments on both sides of the debate about the use of GMOs in food products, primarily about the safety of those who consume it. Anything with GMOs in it is typically excluded from the Whole food challenge and lifestyle.

Sugar products: The rule of thumb here is that if it ends in "ose" and contains any kind of syrup or malt, it's not a good thing to consume.

The bottom line is this: ingredients produced out of a factory do not count as real food. They do not contribute to cellular health and, as such, do not belong in the human body. Cellular health is created when we eat whole foods that do not have anything added to nor taken away from their original forms.

Every single person needs different levels of each food group to thrive and survive. By following and implementing the whole food challenge and lifestyle, you get to pick and choose what combinations and products work for you and your family. You also have to keep in mind that each stage of your life requires different nourishment and "flourishment" needs, so take your age into account as well.

Chapter 4: Persistence Is the Key to Resistance

The Initial Detox

Information overload? No worries. It's really quite simple. The 30-day whole food challenge is all about enacting a lifestyle change, one that you will never regret doing and that will come naturally to you in time.

Let's jump right into the initial Detox. We discussed earlier the importance of detoxifying your body first and foremost, regardless of which diet or regime you want to participate in. You can't build a new house on top of an old and damaged one—you have to first dismantle the old house down to its foundation. It is the same thing with our bodies.

Many programs out there promise unrealistic results under unrealistic timelines, but the truth is, losing weight and changing your lifestyle requires real dedication. As with anything that challenges us, however, those who power through the initial pain to get to the gain will be the ones who'll reap great rewards.

According to the University of Oregon, 95% of dieters report that they gain half if not all of their lost weight back within one to five years. You don't want to be in the 95%. Our first step to ensuring that is to stick to the initial Detox as much as you possibly can to come out at the end of the 30 days with a different mindset—one where you'll be ready to follow through with your actions.

You may be thinking, this is all "easier said than done." It does sound really simple, but let's be honest, changing our eating patterns and even trying to change those of our family, is right up there in difficulty with a Survivor episode. But don't let your busy life, or your family's size and pickiness, distract you from the main goal. It *can* be as easy as it appears.

Starve Your Body the Good Way

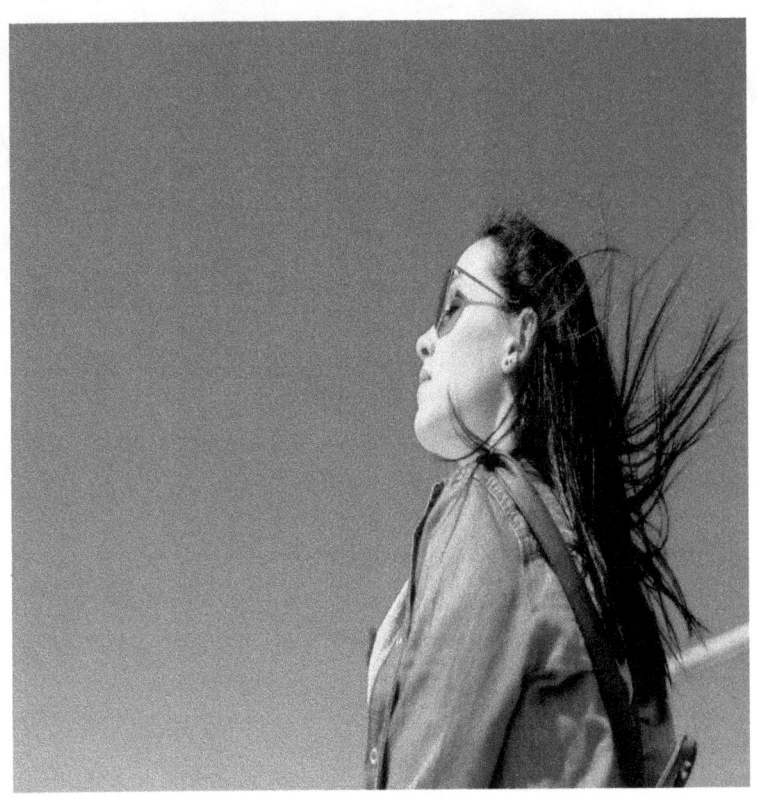

The idea here is to change your mind set during the 30-day Detox and to transform your relationship with the food you eat and buy. This first 30 days is about removing everything that can cause an inflammation in your system. What those items are we discussed in Chapter 3, but to summarize, it's basically anything that had been processed. No alcohol, grains, beans or legumes, dairy products, artificial sweeteners, or sugar is allowed, and certainly nothing that could be labeled as junk food. Instead of those items, go with three organic meals made with whole food ingredients per day.

Before we go any further, please note that we are not doctors. It's important that you also consult a qualified healthcare professional in case your body reacts negatively to sudden, extreme changes to your diet.

When you start your journal during your 30-day Detox, identify how you feel after you have stopped eating these foods. Notice if you have brighter eyes, clearer skin, less chronic pain, more energy, and decreased appetite. Notice all the significant changes and/or improvement in your overall health.

If you have a large family in different age groups, we recommend that you start the Detox by yourself so you can note these changes and get a better idea of how to adjust the diet to better suit the needs, schedule, and makeup of the rest of your family.

How to Remain Persistent in Maintaining Lifetime Habits

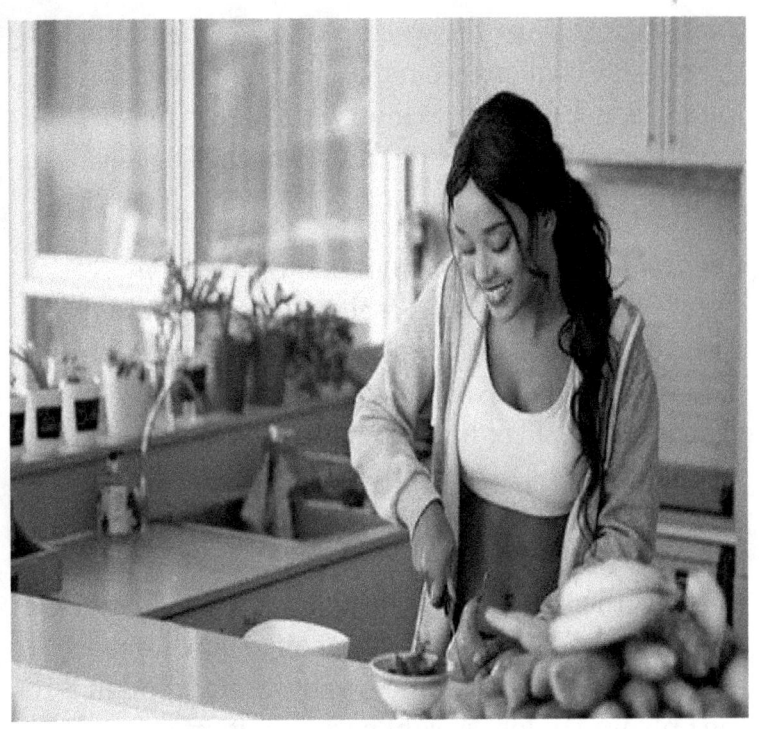

Don't let the terms "whole food" and "organic" scare you off. You may have tasted some tofu before and think that we are talking about eating that for the next 30 days. As tempting as that sounds, we will spare you. Most of the time, what we have found from talking to numerous people is that they are either overcooking their vegetables, which means they're removing the nutrients, or simply under-seasoning them, meaning they fail to bring out the natural flavors.

Try not to be distracted by your busy life, either. We are all swamped and struggling to make the most out of 24 hours in a day, regardless of where we live.

That's just the way the world works. As mentioned, this 30-day challenge is not a diet but a habit-forming foundation for an entire lifestyle. There is only so much overindulgence one can stomach. The idea is to be sensible, healthy, and wise.

Changing what you eat is not enough. You have to start with how you think, feel, buy, and react to the food you eat. A healthy mind and body go hand in hand—you can't have one without the other. Let us have an example of how to change your mind set. Two-thirds of the diets on the market today only focus on the food. They don't get in to *why* you should choose to eat that food. When we take a step back and examine the whys of our eating habits, we'll get to the root cause and can ultimately change how we react and feel through disciplined training and thinking. It's the only way to lose weight and *keep* it off.

If you make a promise to yourself to do X, lose Y, and not eat Z only to end up breaking that promise to your-self, will you hold yourself accountable and haul yourself off to nutrition prison? Most likely not. Nobody likes being lied to, and we certainly shouldn't do it to ourselves. It will only leave us feeling worse. We will discuss creating your own support system later on in this book. For now, please keep that thought about holding yourself accountable in mind.

Chapter 5: Foods You Can Enjoy

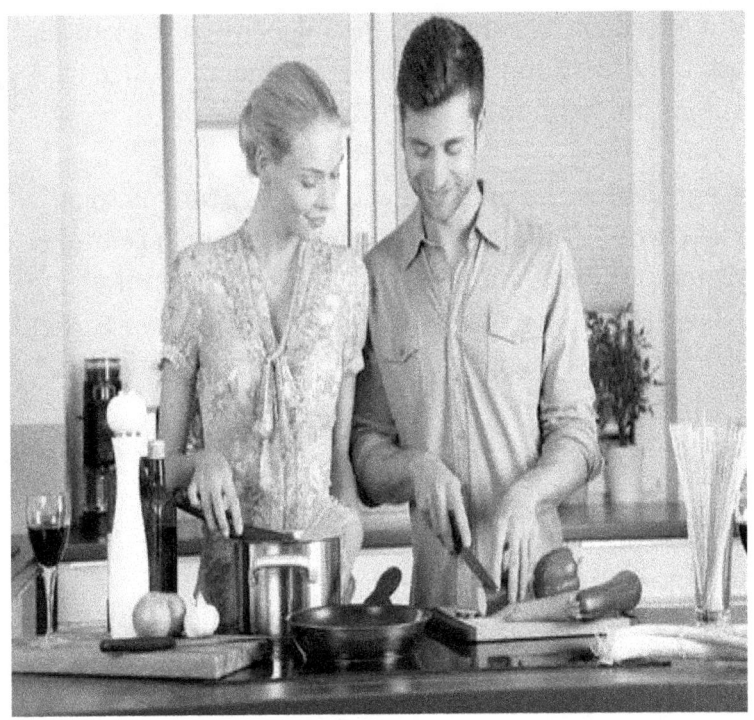

Are you tired of hearing about what you *can't* do and ready to hear what you CAN? Thought so! This is the best part: learning about the whole foods you and your family can enjoy to get into the right mindset and train your palate.

Fruits: There are a lot of people who cook or grill their fruit—the chef Bobby Flay, for one, says it is delicious—but it is still best to eat your fruits raw. Your local supermarket may have seasonal dried fruit, frozen fruits, plenty of canned fruit brands, and these can be a great substitute when your favorite fruits are out of season. Meanwhile, the majority of fruit juices are full of nothing but sugar; it's not a great idea to substitute fresh fruit for fruit juice.

Vegetables: As much as you possibly can, go to a local farmer's market or buy seasonal, fresh produce from your local supermarket. It's even better if you have the space in your home to start your own garden. Prepare these veggies by steaming them lightly. That way, they'll retain their nutrients, color ,and crispness.

Fish: If you can buy local fresh fish, by all means, take advantage of that. As much as possible, avoid buying fish raised on a farm. These particular fish are fed antibiotics to fight off diseases they could contract when kept in close quarters with other fish. They are also easily susceptible to diseases simply from living in unnatural conditions. Fish is always a great source of natural fats.

Nuts: The best type of nuts to consume is whole or raw nuts. Raw peanuts and peanut butter are not what we are referring to here.

Whole Grains: A great option for good cellular health is cooking and eating whole grains like oats, rye, seedless grasses, and rice as well as true whole grains like wheat berries, barley and quinoa, which are gluten-free and high in protein. Each of these whole grains can be cooked and consumed like you would rice, and you can even add them to your salads, soups, and stews, among many others. Whole grains are also great with plain yogurt.

Legumes: If you aren't a fan of seafood, you can use legumes as your source of protein. Eating them raw and when they're in season are the healthiest choices. You can do a lot with legumes because of their versatility. You can add them to dips, put them in soups, or blend and puree them to make sandwich spreads. They go well in casseroles and are great for healthy cell nutrition.

Meat products: This is one of the great benefits of taking the 30-day whole food challenge—meat! As long as the source of meat was grass-fed and free-range, it is acceptable to consume. You want to eat beef from cows that have been fed nothing but grains and/or grass. When animals eat an organic diet, they contain lower fat and are much easier to digest. Remember the food chain—the healthier the prey, the healthier the animals that consume them. It's the same thing with us humans, and it's extremely imperative that we eat for the reason that our bodies were intended to do so: to repair our cells.

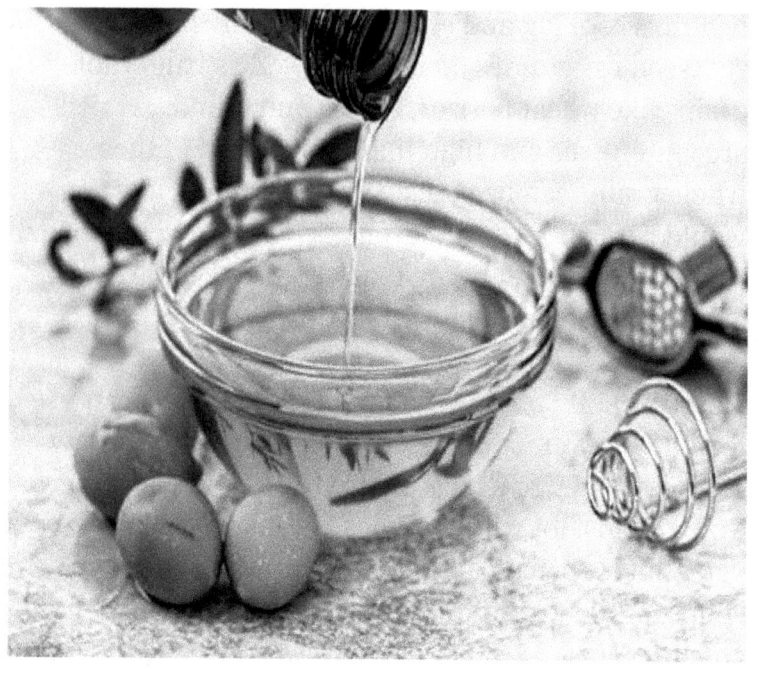

Good fats and oils: It's best to stay away from real butter as much as possible during your challenge and get your necessary good fats from the variety of whole foods you eat. All of the different whole foods we have listed in this guide contain varying amounts of fat content.

If you want to keep track of the whole foods that contain the highest fat content, below is a short list. Do not be afraid to get your fats naturally from the foods you eat as it always results in better health, better moods, and decreased pain and inflammation.

- Use sesame seeds, not sesame oil
- Choose almonds or almond butter instead of almond oil
- Use olives instead of olive oil
- Opt for flax seeds and not flaxseed oil
- Go with avocados and not avocado oil
- Eat soybeans but not soy

For cooking, the best oils to use on the 30-day whole food challenge are sesame oil and coconut oil.You can also substitute extra virgin olive oil as long as the label reads that it is "cold-pressed."It's perfect for salad dressings and for seasoning vegetables.Ghee is also a great option, and it will be discussed further in the next chapter.

Calorie Calculator

While the whole food challenge is strict about not counting calories during the first 30 days, it will be an important part of your meal planning process after your 30-day detox.We've provided a simple online calorie counter that you can use immediately after the initial 30 days have passed.

https://www.calculator.net/calorie-calculator.html

Calorie Calculator

The *Calorie Calculator* can be used to estimate the number of calories a person needs to consume each day. This calculator can also provide some simple guidelines for gaining or losing weight. Use the "metric units" tab if the International System of Units (SI) is preferred.

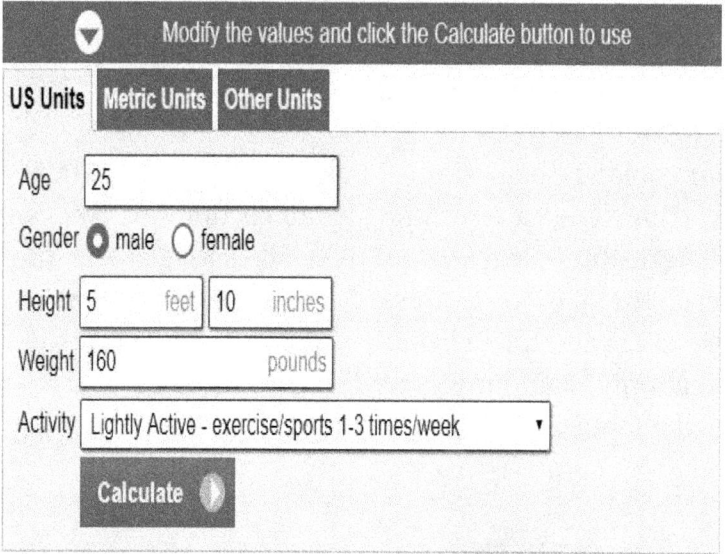

You need **2,361** Calories/day to maintain your weight.
You need **1,861** Calories/day to lose 1 lb per week.
You need **1,361** Calories/day to lose 2 lb per week.
You need **2,861** Calories/day to gain 1 lb per week.
You need **3,361** Calories/day to gain 2 lb per week.

Chapter 6: The 30-Day Challenge

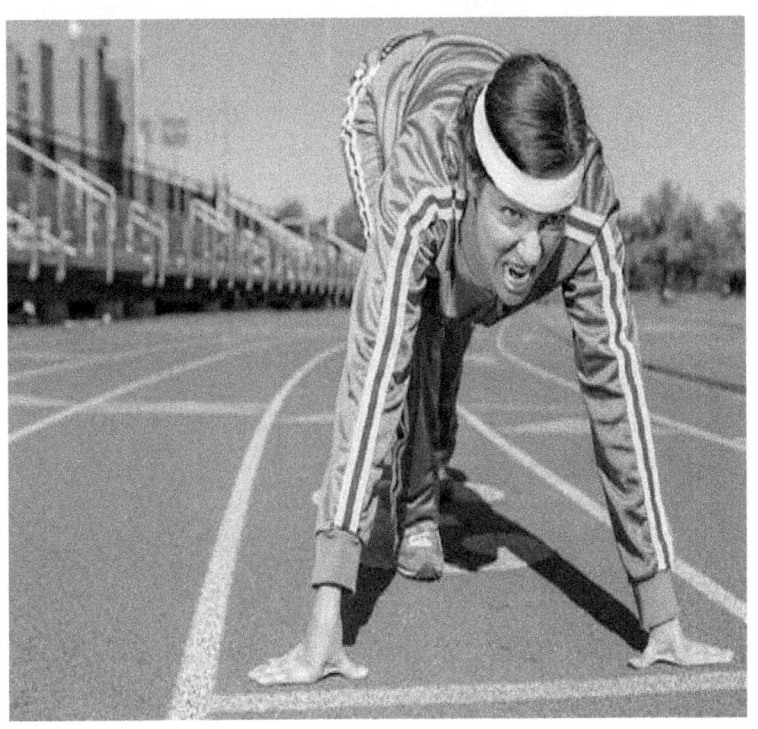

Challenge Accepted!

Congratulations! By this time, we hope you are ready to take into account what we discussed and to accept this challenge fairly and persistently. This will be the turning point in your quest for healthy living and eating. It's now time to make the decision of whether or not this is the right diet for you and/or your family. There are thousands of success stories on the internet from people who are living a whole food lifestyle. They report that they have seen an improvement or found an unofficial cure for the following diseases and ailments:

- Asthma
- Allergies
- High blood pressure
- High cholesterol
- Sinus infections
- Hives
- Skin conditions
- Endometriosis
- PCOS
- Infertility
- Migraines
- Depression
- Bipolar disorder
- Heartburn
- GERD
- Arthritis
- Joint pain
- ADD/ADHD
- Thyroid dysfunction
- Lyme disease
- Fibromyalgia
- Chronic fatigue
- Type 1 diabetes
- Type 2 diabetes
- Lupus
- Leaky gut syndrome
- Crohns
- IBS
- Celiac disease
- Diverticulitis
- Ulcerative colitis

If you are ready to accept the challenge, make the commitment to stick to the plan and follow through until you have rid yourself of your bad eating habits. But just because you make this commitment today, it doesn't mean that you are expected to start dieting immediately. You will need to make the necessary preparations first. Start by clearing out any of the foods you should avoid from your fridge and cabinets. Take a look at the recipes provided in Chapter 8 and make a grocery list of ingredients you will need to pick up at the supermarket.

Sit down and plan your meals for the next 30 days. We've provided a 7-day meal plan to get you started. We've also provided a blank meal plan guide for you to use later on. You will want to include the following in your meal plan: breakfast, lunch, dinner, dessert, and snack.

Now, let's dive into the rules and guidelines of the whole food challenge.

The Whole Food Challenge Rules and Guidelines

I want to start with a small reminder of the foods to avoid during your whole food challenge, most especially during your 30-day Detox. Again, this is not a pick-three menu. We are talking about 100% elimination for at least the first 30 days. This is going to help build your relationship with your food and curb your cravings. It will also help you burn more calories, reduce chronic pain and swelling, improve your mood, and begin cellular repair in your gut.

Again, this is only for the first 30 days... no sweat!

Grains: Avoid corn, millet, sorghum, amaranth, buckwheat, bulgur, sprouted grains, rice, or wheat.

Alcohol: You will want to avoid consuming or cooking with alcohol .Sadly, this even includes vanilla extract, which contains alcohol. Kampuchea tea, meanwhile, is completely acceptable to drink since it contains exceedingly small amounts of alcohol. The main thing to avoid here is the sugars and additives found in fruit juice.

Legumes/Beans: During your first 30 days of Detox, you cannot consume the majority of bean or soy products. This includes tofu, soy sauce, peas, lentils, and even peanuts.

Dairy products: Avoid eating anything with milk, butter, and (especially) cheese.

Junk food: Junk food is a broad category, but remember what we discussed in earlier chapters. If it comes in a package, box, or carton, it's not a good choice. This is part of the mental portion of the healthy eating process and of changing your relationship with the food you eat as you reintroduce them one at a time.

Package label ingredients: If the product label you are reading contains carrageen and, sulfites, or MSG in any form or fashion, please avoid it.

Others: Stay away from sweets, pizza, fast food, French fries, and anything of the like.

Always keep in mind that changing your lifestyle depends on you being disciplined in your choices and following through. Don't just focus on losing weight. Remember that what we eat also affects our moods and behaviors. During this first 30 days, stay focused and, most importantly, *do not* count your calories or use the weighing scale. Measure your weight only once at the beginning so you can see your progress when you weigh yourself again at the end of the 30 days.

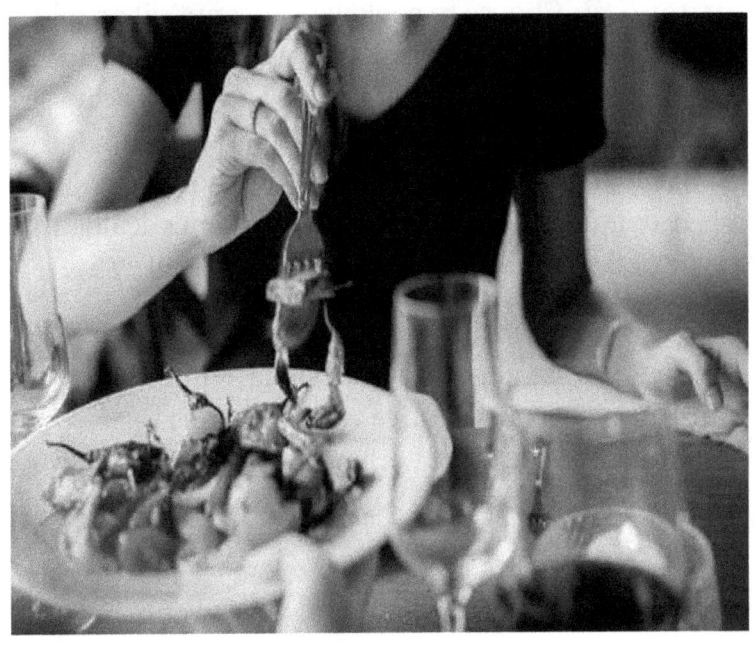

So that we don't leave things on a sour note here, let's discuss a few of the things that get a pass during your whole food challenge.

Drinks: Coffee lovers rejoice—you most certainly can drink your cup of coffee in the morning, but drink it black. Do not add any dairy or artificial sweeteners. You can use any other type of milk, preferably plant-based like coconut milk that does not contain sweeteners.

Nuts/Seeds: You can eat nuts and even seeds, but not peanuts as it's actually a legume.

Butter/Oil: Choose to cook with coconut oil or cold-pressed extra virgin olive oil, but use absolutely *no* butter. Remember, there is a product called ghee which is a clarified butter that originated in India. It's primarily used in South Asia and the Middle East, but it is becoming more commonly used domestically. It is a type of fat that is considered good for healthy cellular reproduction.

Dairy: The one item that you can have in this category is eggs. Be creative when it comes to preparing eggs for meals other than breakfast. They are especially delicious when boiled and added to salads.

Meats: Shellfish of any kind, most types of fish, and any meat that is not processed get a pass. Also, as long as the sausage does not have any preservatives or sugars, you may enjoy that as well. Many turkey sausage varieties offer this choice.

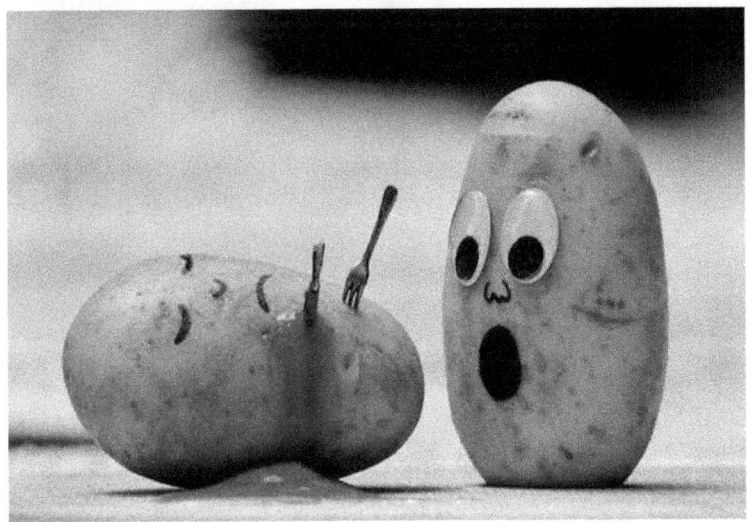

Fruits and vegetables: Fruits must be eaten in moderation. Remember that most fruits have natural sugars in them, and we want to reduce your sugar intake during this critically important 30 days. Eat all vegetables, even potatoes, but make sure they have come in its original brown and round form. French fries are not counted.

Commit!

One of the main reasons that the whole food challenge is one of the easiest to maintain and reap immediate benefits from is that your main goal during those 30 days is to build a relationship with the food you choose to eat. Read those product labels like we have mentioned several times. Do not weigh yourself or count calories at all for the duration of the challenge. Unless you have the time, you do not have to drive 30 miles out of town to visit a "special organic farm"—your supermarket will do just fine. If you have a farmer's market that is close by, that is even better. Most of them can be found on the side of the road or in vacant lots around the city.

If you have a special occasion coming up, you might want to wait until that's over before getting started. We oftentimes use holidays, birthdays, weddings, or anniversaries as an excuse to cheat on our diets. While nobody is going to pop out from under the table and scream at you through a megaphone to drop and give them 30, remember that this is about self-discipline and holding yourself accountable. Every time you cheat, you have to go back to day 1.That's not going to be fun after the second or third time. This cheating and having to start over is what leads many people to give up and move on to some other diet that isn't focused on combining mental health and body fitness into one.

To fully commit to the process, you need to come up with a start date. Without one, our procrastination takes over. It's natural and it happens to the best of us.

How are you going to maintain and keep going so you don't have a slip-up? How can you easily watch your spouse or your co-workers pigging out on pizza and chicken wings without wanting a bite yourself? We recommend that you get a support system in place to help you. Tell your family, friends, co-workers, and social media accounts about what you're doing. Get a journal and a planner and prepare to start building your relationship with food and with a "whole" new you!

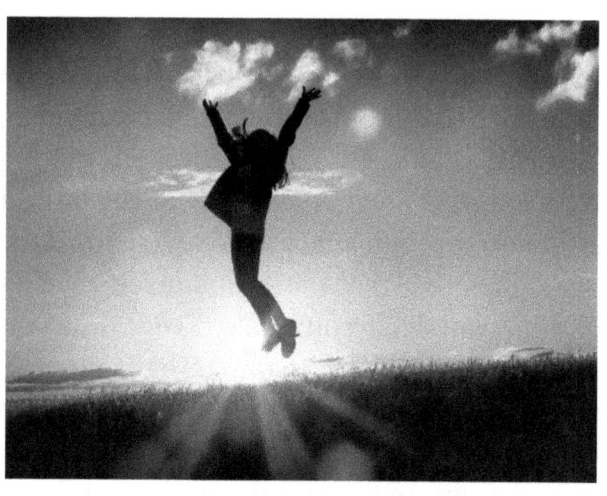

Get Your Support System in Order

No lifestyle change is easy, and trying to do it alone can be especially challenging for many people. Maybe your family setup is not conducive to this type of dieting at the moment; maybe your significant other is not on the same health plane that you are. Whatever the case may be, there are others out there going through the same exact same thing as you. They are there to help you, encourage you, challenge you, and hold you accountable when you can't do it for yourself.

If you do have a great support system at home, capitalize on that! Use your friends and family's love and encouragement to help you be successful and disciplined. They do not have to go on the diet, too. They can simply be there to give you the push you need. If you belong to any organizations or charities, other members might be willing to support you as well. Explain to people why you are choosing to do this, why you want their support particularly, and then get to the point—come right out and ask them if they will be your support system while you change your relationship with the food you eat. Most people will say yes, but make sure you are choosing wisely.

We've seen many a Friday night (with pizza and a cold one) take out dedicated whole food challengers and send them back down the slide to day 1. Never a good feeling. Choose someone who will take your vision and goals, treat them as their own, and actually hold you accountable. You don't want to elicit the support of someone who will enable you or turn a blind eye if you slide down that slippery baked goods slope.

Behavioral changes only happen with consistency. We cannot, unfortunately, click our heels three times and magically be the size we want to be. We also can't do something for 9 days, take 2 weeks off, then go full steam for 12 days before taking 21 days off. It doesn't work that way. Asking for help is not something to be avoided, and you shouldn't be ashamed to do it. Having the courage to do it is actually a sign of strength.

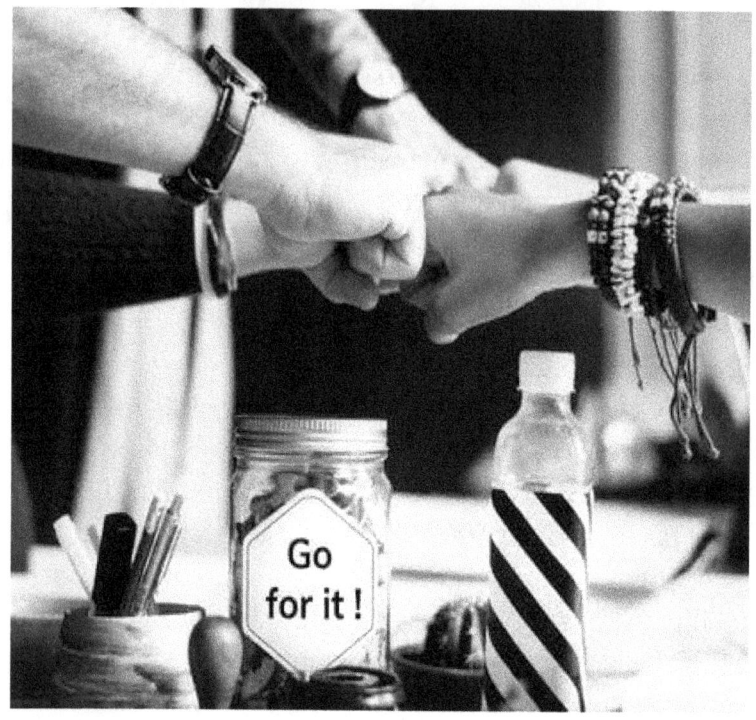

Find a compatible diet buddy to inspire you. Whether you choose someone who you can meet up with in person or prefer the anonymity of an internet buddy, the key factor is that whoever you choose has to want the same thing you do .It also really isn't that important *how* you communicate or what methods you use. The goal is to take time to hear each other's struggles and celebrate the successes together. It's not always about having someone standing over you as you choose what to eat and how you eat it.

Social media is a force to be reckoned with when it comes to accountability in the diet world Facebook is notorious for having thousands of groups that encourage you to participate. There are no age, gender, or diet restrictions in some of the groups; it's a group dedicated to supporting each other no matter what program you are on. The *#fbbgirls* by Anna Victoria is a prime example of women just supporting other women on their journey to a healthier lifestyle. Many people we talk to find comfort, accountability, and even inspiration from these online support groups that are made up of people who can identify with others who are facing similar struggles. You've got this! *You've got this!*

Read on to see the 7-day meal plan to help you kick-start your 30-day whole food challenge with a bang!

7-Day Meal Plan – Planning for Success

Day 1 Mon	Day 2 Tues	Day 3 Wed	Day 4 Thurs	Day 5 Fri	Day 6 Sat	Day 7 Sun
Breakfast	**Breakfast**	**Breakfast**	**Breakfast**	**Breakfast**	**Breakfast**	**Breakfast**
2 Egg Cups ½ Cup Sweet Potato Hash ¼ Avocado 1 Cup Mixed Berries Green Tea	2 Egg Cups ½ Cup Sweet Potato Hash ¼ Avocado 1 Cup Mixed Berries Green Tea	2 Egg Cups ½ Cup Sweet Potato Hash ¼ Avocado 1 Cup Mixed Berries Green Tea	2 Egg Cups ½ Cup Sweet Potato Hash ¼ Avocado 1 Cup Mixed Berries Green Tea	2 Egg Cups ½ Cup Sweet Potato Hash ¼ Avocado 1 Cup Mixed Berries Green Tea	2 Eggs Cups 3 Slices Bacon ¼ Avocado 1 Cup Arugula 1 Cup Mixed Berries Green Tea	2 Eggs Frittata Chicken Apple Sausage ¼ Avocado 1 Cup Mixed Berries Green Tea
Lunch	**Lunch**	**Lunch**	**Lunch**	**Lunch**	**Lunch**	**Lunch**
Salad Jar Kale, Shredded Carrots, Radish, Cherry Tomato 6 oz Grilled Chicken 1 Tbsp Olive Oil	Salad Jar Kale, Shredded Carrots, Radish, Cherry Tomato 6 oz Grilled Chicken 1 Tbsp Olive Oil	Salad Jar Kale, Shredded Carrots, Radish, Cherry Tomato 6 oz Grilled Chicken 1 Tbsp Olive Oil	Salad Jar Kale, Shredded Carrots, Radish, Cherry Tomato 6 oz Grilled Chicken 1 Tbsp Olive Oil	Salad Jar Kale, Shredded Carrots, Radish, Cherry Tomato 6 oz Grilled Chicken 1 Tbsp Olive Oil	Tuna Salad Boats Peppers 1 Tbsp Mayo Sweet Potato Fries	Leftover Lemon Garlic Chicken Thigh Lettuce Wraps 1 Tbsp Mayo Diced Pepper
Dinner	**Dinner**	**Dinner**	**Dinner**	**Dinner**	**Dinner**	**Dinner**
Grass Fed Burger Kale Bun Guacamole Salad	Turkey Chili Spaghetti Squash Salad	Salmon Roasted Brussel Sprouts Salad	Leftover Turkey Chili Spaghetti Squash Salad	Lemon Garlic Chicken Thighs Grilled Asparagus Salad	Grilled Rib eye Steak Butter Lettuce Salad	Grilled Chicken Breast Grilled Veggies Salad
Snack	**Snack**	**Snack**	**Snack**	**Snack**	**Snack**	**Snack**
Sliced Apple 1 Tbsp Almond Butter Iced Green Tea	Pear 15 Raw Cashews Iced Green Tea	Sliced Apple 1 Tbsp Cashew Butter Iced Green Tea	Pear 3 Slices Prosciutto Iced Green Tea	Sliced Apple 15 Almonds Iced Green Tea	Sliced Apple 3 Slices Prosciutto Iced Green Tea	Sliced Apple 1 Tbsp Almond Butter Iced Green Tea

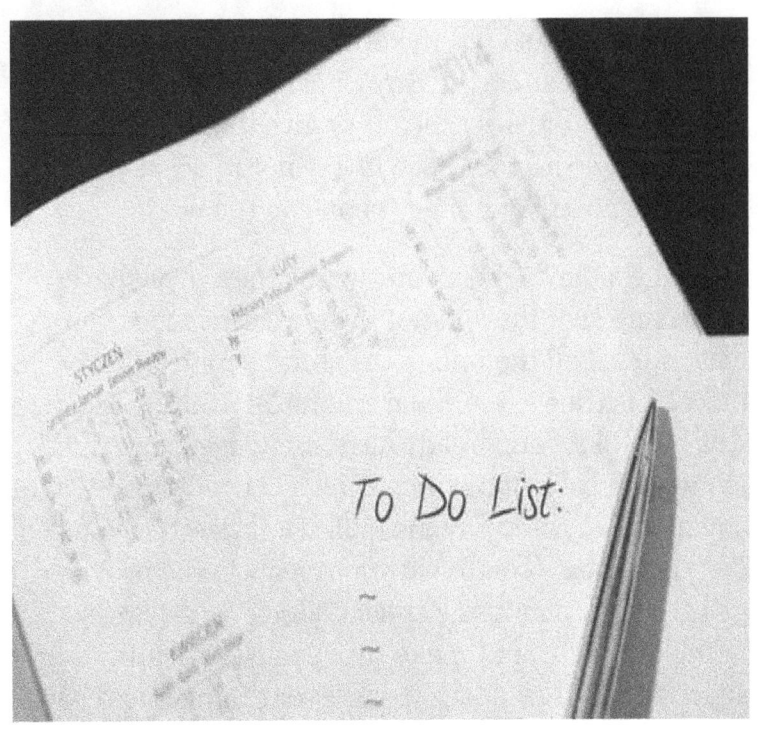

Implement and Repeat

We briefly discussed in earlier chapters the importance of planning in this process. To be successful at anything, a well-thought-out plan of action is always best, and dieting is no exception.

As mentioned before, the first thing you want to do is to get rid of all the foods you cannot have .If you are the only one in your family who is doing the diet, you will want to avoid an uprising by giving them a space to store food away from yours. It is important that you aren't tempted, so put the others' food out of your reach. If you can, avoid throwing the food in the trash. Take it to a homeless shelter or give it to someone in your family who could use it. Try not to waste it when there are plenty of hungry people in the world.

Just as you have given your family their own space, make sure that they do not invade yours. Once you have moved all the unhealthy stuff to some other place, it is time to sit down and make your grocery list .It's helpful if you already have some meals in mind, along with each of the ingredients you will need. Take advantage of the 7-day meal plan to kick-start your diet, and then write down your meals in the provided 30-day meal planner. Replace "Sides" with "Snacks" in the template, and make sure you eat a healthy snack in between meals to curb your hunger and bad cravings.

Once you have removed all the foods you cannot have, made space for your family's food, reviewed the recipes, and made a list of ingredients, it's time to go shopping! Things don't start and end at the supermarket. You know your individual lifestyle and circumstances. Think of everything that could possibly prevent you from doing what you need to do on this 30-day whole food challenge and come up with a strategy on how to combat or overcome them.

Here are a couple examples that you can use as a guide:

Wedding/Anniversary party: If someone bothers you about not eating cake, simply tell them something along the lines of "I'm in the process of reducing my sugar intake to document how it affects my mood .See how pleasant I am right now? That might change if you keep offering me cake..."

Running late: Let's be honest here- Who has not run late at some point in their life and settled for a fast food burger or a gas station abomination to keep your stomach from embarrassing you in your meeting? Plan at the start of each day to prevent that from ever happening again, for overrun conference calls, PTA meetings after work, soccer practice for the twins, or ballet lessons for your daughter, you can learn all about how to pack kale chips, raw veggies, and/or fruit as a travel snack daily instead of going for unhealthy options because you had no choice. Don't be a repeat "day 1-er"!

30 Day Meal Plan Template (Replace Side with snack!)

Whole 30 Meal Planner

	Day 1	Day 2	Day 3	Day 4	Day 5
Breakfast					
Lunch					
Dinner					
Side					
	Day 6	Day 7	Day 8	Day 9	Day 10
Breakfast					
Lunch					
Dinner					
Side					
	Day 11	Day 12	Day 13	Day 14	Day 15
Breakfast					
Lunch					
Dinner					
Side					
	Day 16	Day 17	Day 18	Day 19	Day 20
Breakfast					
Lunch					
Dinner					
Side					
	Day 21	Day 22	Day 23	Day 24	Day 25
Breakfast					
Lunch					
Dinner					
Side					
	Day 26	Day 27	Day 28	Day 29	Day 30
Breakfast					
Lunch					
Dinner					
Side					

Chapter 7: Kitchen Essentials

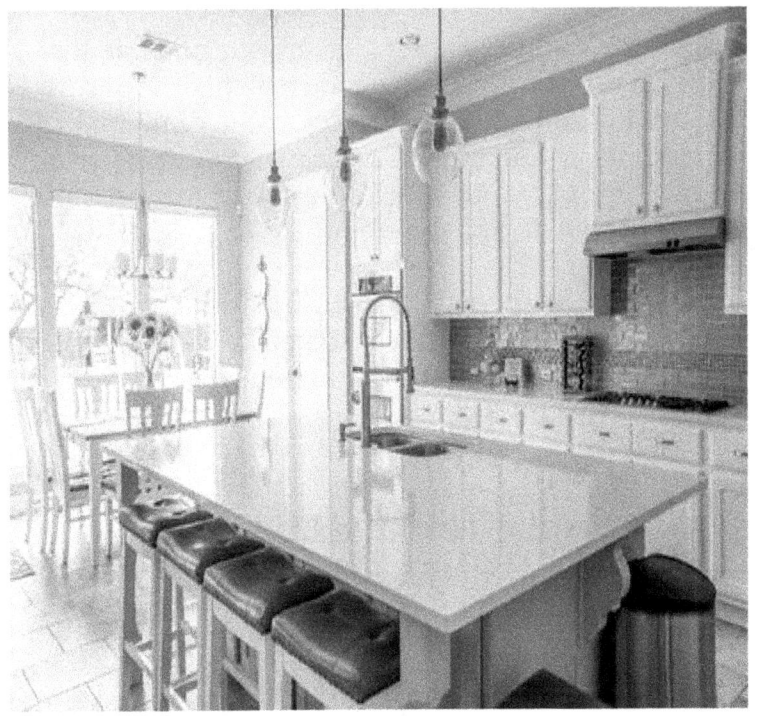

Key Ingredients Needed on Hand

Fruit bowl: Keep a bowl of fruit on the counter. Ignore those junk food cravings and simply grab a fresh piece of fruit when you need something to munch on. Pears, bananas, apples, and Clementine's are great additions to a fruit bowl.

Spices galore: A complete set of spices is the key to helping you enjoy the food you prepare at home. You can also make your own unique house blend by mixing together your favorite flavors and spices.

A well-stocked freezer: One of your best friends while on the 30-day whole food challenge is your freezer .Instead of ice cream and frozen dinners, bag up fresh fruits and veggies in snack and dinner-size portions for easy retrieval. You can keep your seafood and meats portioned in freezer bags as well.

Flavored water: Soda and sugary drinks are always the hardest to bid farewell to. To make water a bit more flavorful, try adding cucumbers, berries, lemons, and herbs like mint.

Kitchen Utensils Every Home Needs

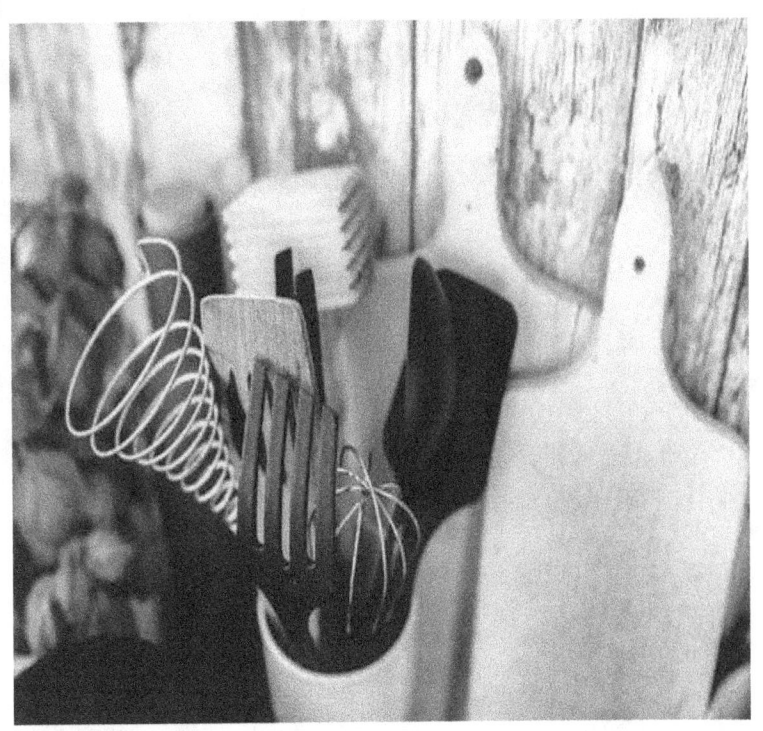

Organize your kitchen for success and make sure that it has all the tools you'll need to have a successful dieting experience. For starters, keep a blender, a whisk, containers with lids, and plenty of baggies.

Chapter 8: Whole Food Recipes for a "Whole" New You

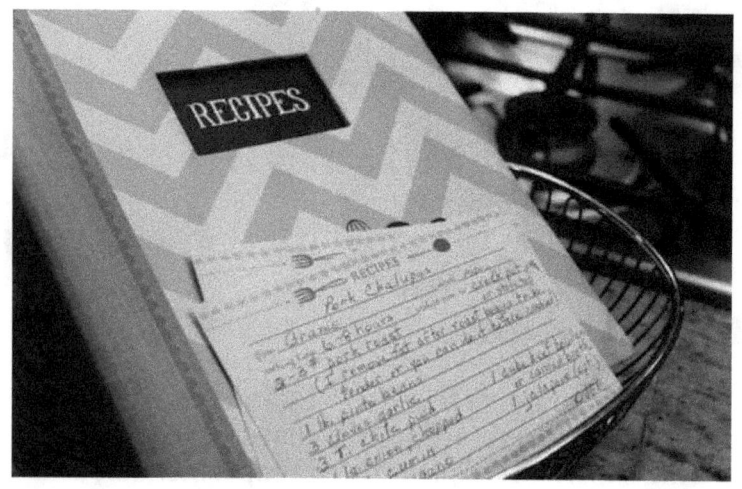

Breakfast Recipes

Try these delicious breakfast recipes to keep building your relationship with whole foods and maintain the integrity of your chosen lifestyle. Enjoy!

Breakfast Bowl with Zucchini Noodles

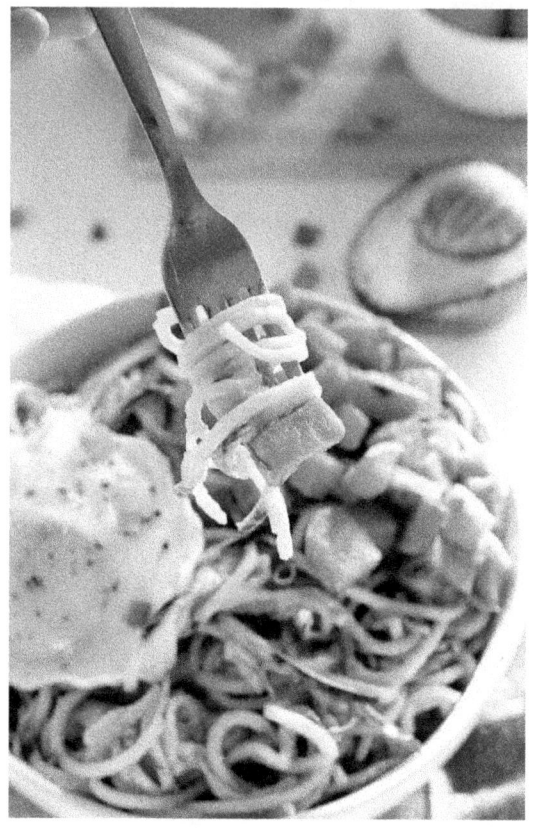

Total Prep & Cooking Time: 30 Minutes
Yields: 2 Servings
Author: The Almond Eater

What's in it:

- Zucchini (1 large piece)
- Avocado (½)
- Olive oil (¼ cup)

- Water (2 tbsp.)
- Garlic cloves (1-2)
- Sweet potatoes (2 whole)
- Eggs (2 large)
- Green onion (2 tbsp.)
- Salt and pepper as desired

How it's made:

1. First, cut and peel the sweet potatoes into ¼-inch cubes. Heat up the oil, cook the potatoes unti lthey're tender, stirring every so often.

2. Chop off the ends of the zucchini and peel off the skin. If you have a spiralizer, you will want to use it to create your noodles.

3. To create the cream, put the avocado, olive oil, garlic, and water in a mixer, blender, or food processor; set it to the pulse setting .Depending on your preference, you might want to add a little more oil to keep it wet and have it mixed properly.

4. Once it's blended well, pour it over the noodles and mix well; when the potatoes are done with a slightly brown and crusted exterior, place them over the noodles.

5. Finally, you will cook your eggs in the exact skillet you cooked the potatoes to pick up those

delicious bits of goodness at the bottom of the pan. Once the egg is cooked to your desired taste, place the eggs atop the noodles and potatoes, then sprinkle everything with green onion. Get ready to eat a delicious, healthy breakfast.

Apple and Cinnamon Hot Cereal

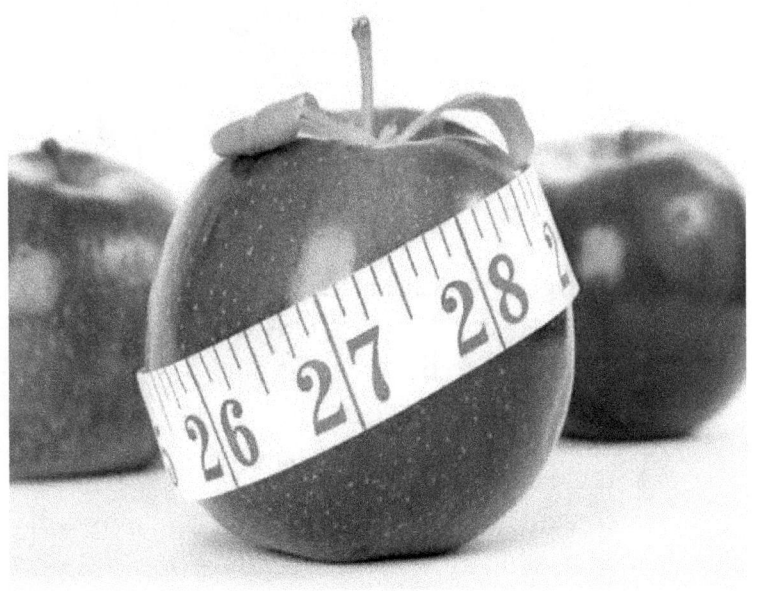

Total Prep & Cooking Time: 10 minutes
Yields: 4 Servings

What's in it:

- Raw almonds whole (½ cup)
- Raw cashews whole (½ cup)
- Raw walnuts (¼ cup)
- Coconut flakes, unsweetened (⅓ cup)
- Banana (1 ripe)
- Egg yolk (1; optional)
- Ghee (1 tbsp.)
- Apple (1 medium; bite-size pieces)

- Ground nutmeg (⅛ tsp.)
- Pure coconut milk (1 ¾ cups)
- Ground cinnamon (2 tbsp.)
- Raisins (½ cup)

How it's made:

1. In a large or medium sized bowl, combine the nuts and coconut flakes. Only use filtered water and add that to the bowl; be sure to completely cover the nuts and coconut.

2. Add a dash of salt and completely cover the bowl with a paper towel or plate. The nuts will need to soak for at least 7-8 hours or overnight.

3. After the allotted time, drain the nuts and coconut flakes. Be sure to completely rinse them until you see clear water running off.

4. Put the nuts and coconut flakes in a mixer. Add the egg yolk (optional) and banana that's been sliced into pieces.

5. Pulse the mixture until it looks like a finely ground nut meal. Be certain to get all the way down the bowl to have an even texture. Remove bowl from food processor and set aside.

6. Add your ghee to a skillet and heat on medium temperature. Put in the chopped apple and

nutmeg and proceed to cook the apples until they become fork-tender.

7. Combine the coconut milk, vanilla, cinnamon and raisins, and the banana-nut meal mixture you just made. Blend them together thoroughly.

8. Bring the hot cereal to a slow simmer and proceed to cook for an additional 5-6 minutes or until your cereal has a thick and creamy texture.

Whole30 Breakfast Bowl

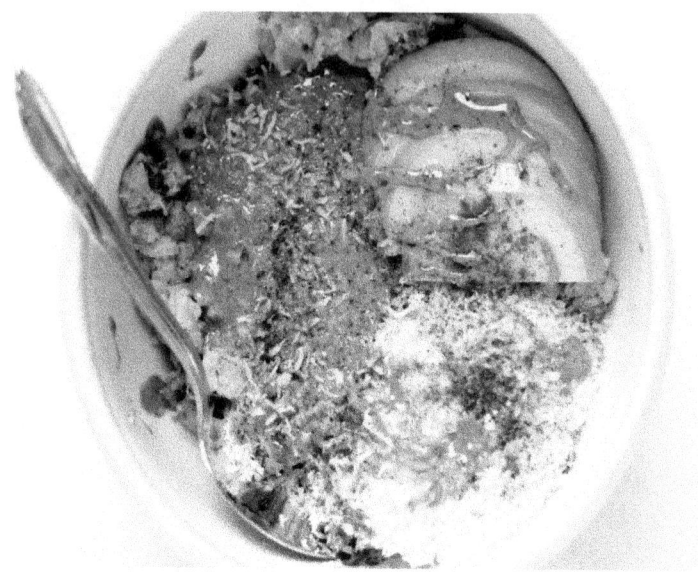

Total Prep & Cooking Time: 15 Minutes
Yields: 1 Serving

What's in it:

- Medium banana (1 ripe)
- Eggs (2)
- Vanilla bean powder (1 tsp.)
- Green apple, sliced (¼ cup)
- Almond butter (1-2 tbsp.)
- Dried coconut flakes (1-2 tbsp.)
- Cinnamon (1 tsp.)
- Coconut oil

How it's made:

1. Mash the ripe banana and mix with the eggs and the vanilla powder in a medium bowl. Do not worry if the batter is lumpy.

2. Grease a hot skillet or pan with the coconut oil and preheat your oven on medium heat. Add in the batter and, with a spatula, continue to stir. At the same time, mash the mixture.

3. When it's done cooking, take the mixture out of the skillet and put it into a clean bowl. You can top it with a fresh piece of fruit of your choice. Add almond butter, cinnamon, and even coconut flakes, if desired.

Simple Breakfast Salad

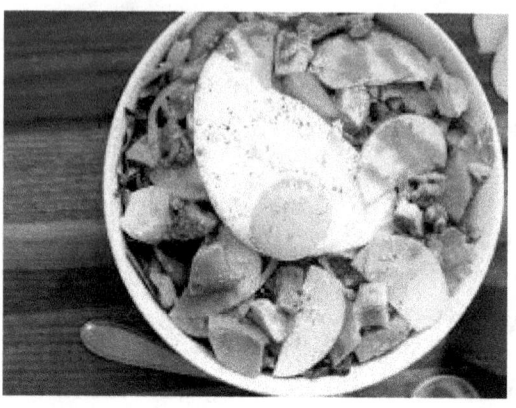

Total Prep & Cooking Time: 5 Minutes
Yields: 1 Serving

What's in it:

- Arugula (1 cup)
- Veggies (1 cup of your favorite leftover or fresh veggies)
- Italian sausage, sliced (1)
- Egg (1)
- Sauerkraut or pickled vegetables (1 cup)
- Hot sauce, for serving

How it's made:

1. Cook the sliced sausage in a medium to high heat skillet for approximately 3 minutes. Make sure to brown it on both sides.

2. After you have flipped the sausage once, add a cracked egg to the same skillet. Cook it for at least 5 minutes but be sure the yolk is still runny; this is essentially your salad dressing.

3. While you wait for the egg to cook, go ahead and put the rest of the ingredients in a microwave-safe dish to warm them up.

4. Add the pickled veggies or sauerkraut to the egg and sausage and, if you like your food spicy, go ahead and add your hot sauce as well. Enjoy lunch for breakfast!

Chia and Banana Pudding

Total Prep & Cooking Time: 35 Minutes
Yields: 6 ½-cup Servings for Freezing

What's in it:

- Water (1 cup)
- Chia seeds (2 1/2 tbsp.)
- Ripe bananas (2)
- Fat-free coconut milk (1 cup)
- Ground cinnamon (1/2 tsp.)
- Dash of salt

How it's made:

Prep

1. In a jar or bowl with a very tight and secure lid, add the chia seeds and water.
2. Shake the mixture until all the chia seeds are incorporated into the water.
3. Put this to the side for about 30 minutes, but keep shaking on occasion to break up lumps and to keep the seeds from settling to the bottom.

To Make the Pudding

1. Combine the coconut milk and the bananas in a blender and run on the pulse setting.
2. Pour the mixture into a bowl, making sure you scrape out the sides of the blender bowl.
3. Add your dry ingredients and refrigerate until it sets. Serve this cold.
4. You can put this into individual containers in single-serving portions and have a week's worth of breakfast.

Oatmeal with No Oats and Zucchini

Total Prep & Cooking Time: 10 minutes
Yields: 1 Serving (Large)

What's in it:

- Egg whites (3/4 cup)
- Unsweetened vanilla almond milk (3/4 cup)
- Ground flaxseed (1 1/2 tbsp.)
- Ripe banana (1/2 large; mashed)
- Zucchini (1/2; grated)
- Cinnamon (1/2 tsp.)

How it's made:

1. In a medium-sized bowl, combine the mashed banana and the zucchini; set it to the side.

2. Over medium heat in a small-sized saucepan, combine egg whites and almond milk, then add the flaxseed and stir until the mixture begins to thicken. Keep scraping the sides of the pan so the mixture doesn't stick.

3. Next, add the banana-zucchini mixture and keep stirring as the oatmeal begins to thicken. It is important that you do not leave or walk away.

4. Add the cinnamon, turn down the heat, and keep stirring until it reaches the desired thickness.

5. If you prefer, you can add your favorite toppings like fruit, nut butter, or even unsweetened corn.

Sweet Potato Mash

Total Prep & Cooking Time: 25 Minutes
Yields: 6 Servings

What's in it:

- Sweet potatoes, peeled (2 pounds)
- Apples or unsweetened applesauce (1/2 pound)
- A pinch of sea salt
- Ghee optional (1 tbsp.)

How it's made:

1. Start by preheating the oven to 400°F. Next, take some parchment paper and line the inside of a baking sheet.

2. Let the potatoes roast in the oven for about an hour. Take them out of the oven and let them cool.

3. Peel the skins off the sweet potatoes. Mash the potatoes well until it's to your desired consistency; you can also use a food processor.

Potato Scramble & Hot Chilies (Optional)

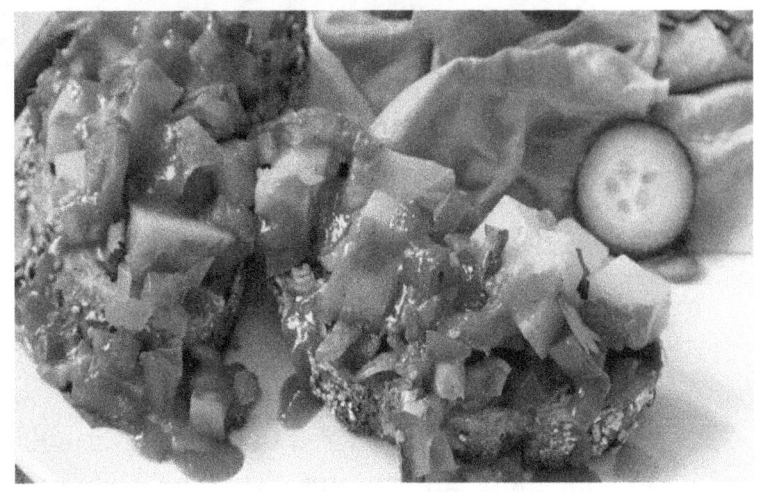

Total Prep & Cooking Time: 35 Minutes
Yields: 1 serving

What's in it:

- Chopped red onion (½ cup)
- Yellow mustard (3 tbsp.)
- Ground allspice (¼ tsp.)
- Finely chopped and seeded jalapeno pepper (1 ½ tsp.)
- Clean potatoes (any, cut into ½ cubes)
- Sea salt
- Tomatoes (1 cup)
- Finely chopped cilantro (½ cup)

- Lime juice (3 tbsp.)
- Whole-grain bread, toasted (6 slices)
- (Optional) hot chilies

How it's made:

1. First, combine a cup of water with the onion, mustard, jalapeno, and allspice in a skillet over medium heat. Cover and cook until you can see through the onions, which will take about 10 minutes.

2. Add the diced potatoes, salt to your liking, and add one more cup of water. Bring the heat to a high setting, then cover and let it cook.Only stir it once or twice during the cooking time(5 minutes each time).

3. Reduce the heat to medium and keep it covered until you can stick a fork through the potatoes, which typically takes 15 minutes.

4. To serve, toast your bread and top with the cooked scramble.Before you serve it, add the remaining ingredients with the hot chili being optional.

Lime, Honeydew, and Vegetable Smoothie

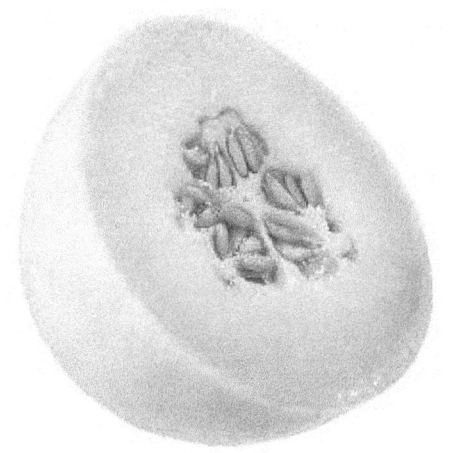

Total Prep & Cooking Time: 5 Minutes
Yields: 2 Servings

What's in it:

- Honeydew (2 cups)
- Bananas (2)
- Lime juice (1 lime)
- Spinach (1 cup)
- Cucumber (1/4, cut)
- Water (1 cup)
- Ice (if needed; 1 cup)

How it's made:

1. Mix everything together in your blender until all the ingredients are combined

2. Serve it cold and enjoy!

Breakfast Salad: BLT Style

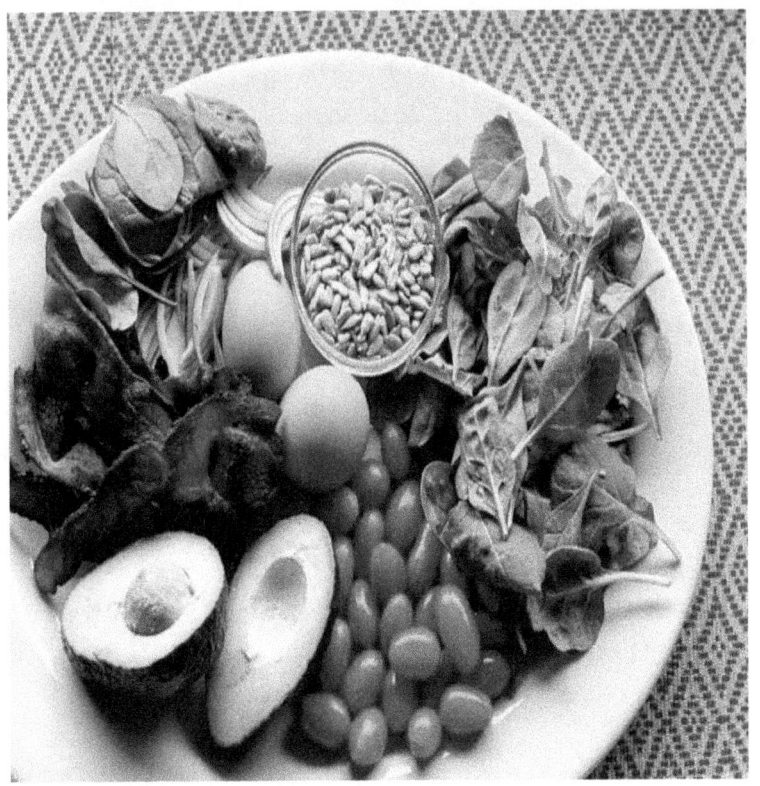

Total Prep & Cooking Time: 10 Minutes
Yields: 2 Servings

What's in it:

- Greens (2 pounds, fresh)
- Red onion, diced (1/4)
- Tomato, seeded and diced (1 large)
- Roasted sunflower seeds (1/3 cup)

- Bacon, chopped and cooked (6 pieces)
- Thinly sliced avocado (1)
- Soft-boiled eggs (2)
- Salt & pepper as desired

To Make the Dressing

- Olive oil (1/4 cup)
- Apple cider vinegar (3 tbsp.)
- Dijon mustard (1 tbsp.)
- Lemon juice (1 lemon)

How it's made:

1. In an adequate-sized bowl, combine your bag of greens with the onion, tomato, sunflower seeds and bacon.

2. Put your salad dressing components in a mason jar. Place the lid on the jar and shake until the dressing is thoroughly combined.

3. Pour your dressing over the salad and mix it thoroughly with your greens Don't be afraid to use your hands.

4. Boil your eggs for 6 minutes and transfer to a bowl of ice water to halt the cooking. When the eggs are cooled, peel, slice, and serve them on top of the salad with some creamy avocado slices.

Salmon Frittatas

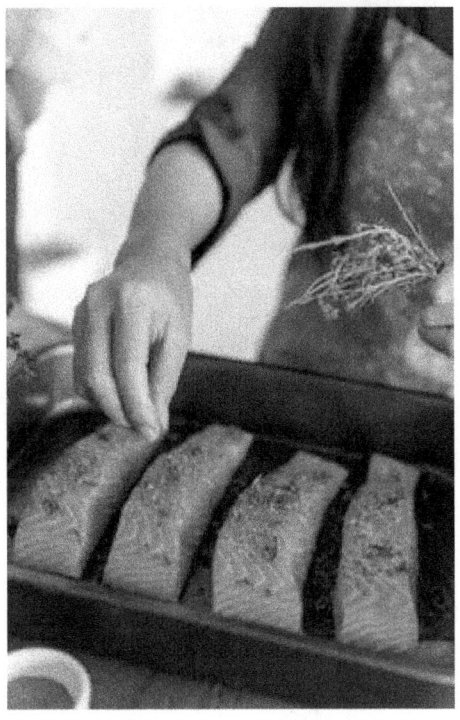

Total Prep & Cooking Time: 45 Minutes
Yields: 6 Servings

What's in it:

- Salmon (1.5 pounds)
- Eggs (10)
- Onion (1/2, small)

- Cooking oil (2 tbsp.)
- Chopped dill (1 tbsp.)
- Chopped capers (1 tbsp.)
- Chopped chives (1 tsp)
- Dill mayo
- Salt and pepper

How it's made:

1. Begin by preheating the oven to 375°F.

2. Take out a large skillet or frying pan and heat up your oil on medium setting.

3. Cut up the salmon in smaller-sized pieces. To your taste, add salt and pepper to each side of the salmon.

4. Once the oil is hot enough, slowly put in the salmon fillets with the skin down. Cook for about 5 minutes or until it's cooked about two-thirds of the way and is no longer sticking to the pan. We do not recommend trying to flip it or remove it from the pan before this point. If you do, it will stick to the pan and you won't get your crispy skin

5. Flip the salmon over and continue cooking for 3 minutes until it is completely cooked through.

6. Lightly grease a baking dish with ghee to further prevent sticking.

7. In a new bowl, whisk the eggs, dill, capers, chives, and a dash of salt and pepper.

8. Crumble the salmon into big pieces and place them in a lightly greased baking dish; pour in your egg mixture.

9. Make sure the egg is evenly coated over the salmon and bake in the oven on 375°F for at least 30 minutes or until the center is dry.

10. Make sure to let the salmon rest for at least 10 minutes before cutting and serving. For added flavor, you can garnish with dill mayo.

Shakshuka with Brussels Sprouts and Spinach

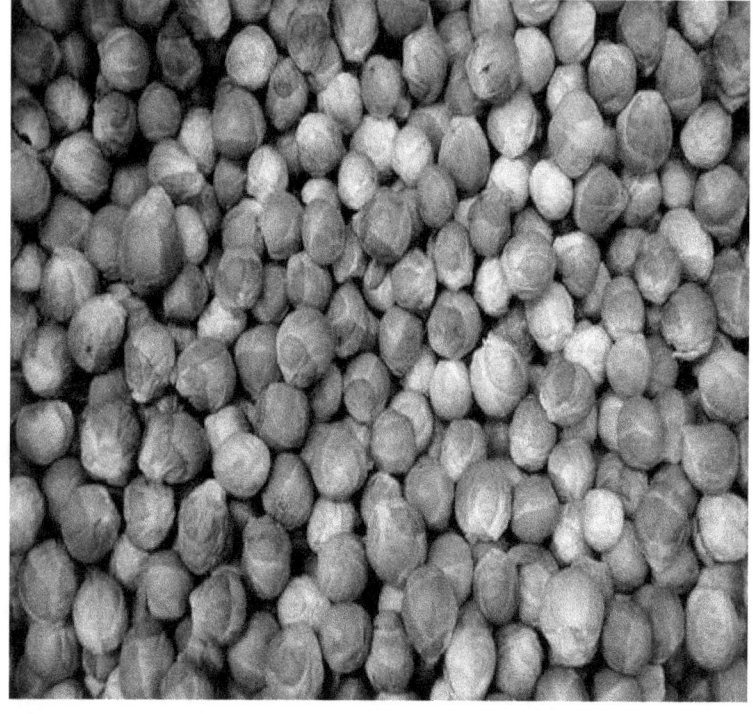

Total Prep & Cooking Time: 40 Minutes
Yields: 4 Servings

What's in it:

- Olive oil (2 tbsp.)
- Onion, diced (½, medium)
- Garlic (4 cloves)
- Brussels sprouts, shaved or finely sliced (2 cups)
- Zucchini, grated (1)
- Cumin (1 tsp.)

- Salt (½ tsp.)
- Pepper (¼ tsp.)
- Fresh cilantro, chopped (¼ cup)
- Baby spinach (2 cups, packed)
- Eggs (4 large)
- Avocado (optional garnish; 1 large)

How it's made:

1. Start by preheating your oven. It needs to be at 375°F.
2. In a medium frying pan or skillet, heat up the olive oil and cook the onions for 5 minutes or until you can see through them. After 5 minutes, you can add the garlic and cook for 1 additional minute.
3. Add the Brussels sprout. When you can fork them, add the zucchini and spices and cook for an additional minute while stirring.
4. Add the spinach after the veggies are completely cooked; stir it in until it wilts. Pat the mixture down evenly all around and then add the raw eggs on top.
5. Put the pan in the oven and cook for at least 8 minutes or until the eggs have cooked as desired.
6. Top with the avocado for each serving (optional).

Chicken, Sausage & Egg Bake

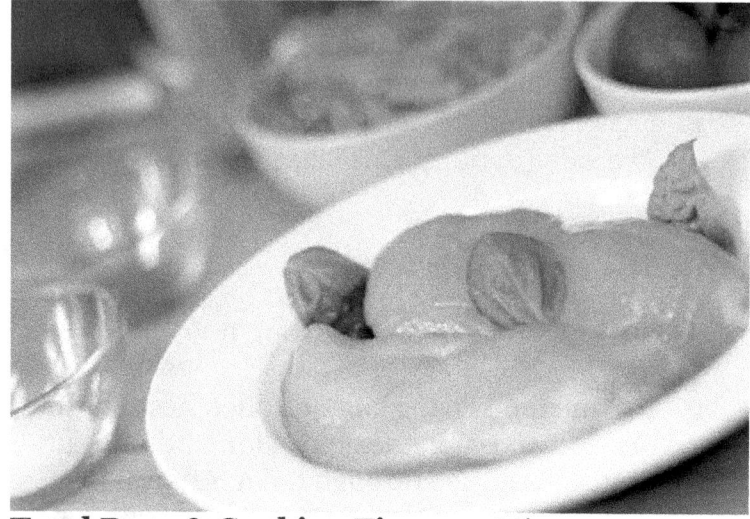

Total Prep & Cooking Time: 45 Minutes
Yields: 6 Servings

What's in it:

- Diced vegetables (choose your 4 favorites)
- Chicken apple sausage (2 links, cut in slices)
- Eggs (2 large)
- Ghee (4 tbsp.)
- Dash of salt and pepper

How it's made:

1. Your oven will need to be set at 350°F to preheat.
2. Cube and dice your favorite veggies; make sure they are completely rinsed and dried. If frozen, make sure they are completely thawed and drained.

3. Use your ghee to coat the bottom of a 9×12 glass baking dish by melting it first in a skillet over the stove. Once the ghee has melted, add your veggies to soften them and a dash of salt and pepper to taste.
4. Add your chicken apple sausage and continue cooking for at least 5 minutes.
5. While that is cooking, begin cracking your eggs. When the vegetables are done, add the eggs into the greased baking dish and cook for 30 minutes or until the edges have turned brown.

Almond Butter & Strawberry Smoothie

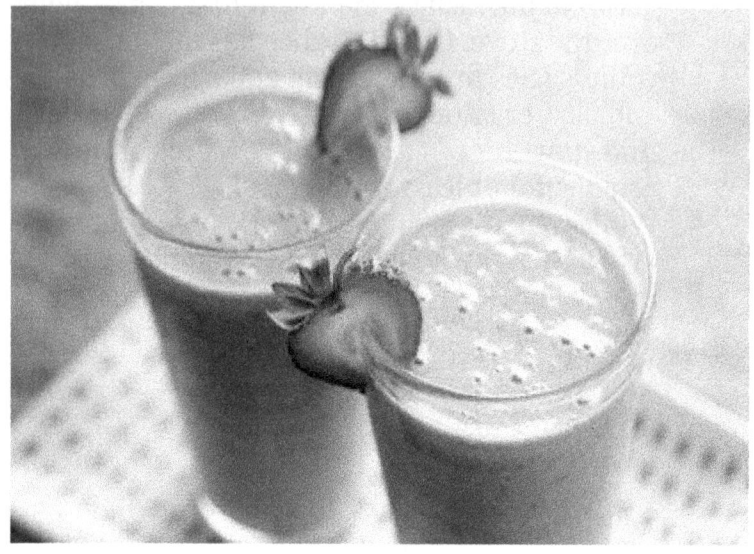

Total Prep & Cooking Time: 5 Minutes
Yields: 1 Cup

What's in it:

- Ice cubes (4 whole)
- Strawberries (8 ounces)
- Unsweetened almond milk (1 cup)
- Smooth almond butter (2 tbsp.)

How it's made:

1. Place all four ice cubes into the blender and completely blend until no chunks remain.
2. Add the fruit, milk, and butter and blend again until a smooth texture has been achieved.
3. Pour and enjoy a healthy drink!

Kale Quiche with Sweet Potato Crust

Total Prep & Cooking Time: 1 hour
Yields: 4 Servings

What's in it:

- Sweet potatoes (2 medium)
- Sweet onion (1/2)
- Kale (6 stalks)
- Broccoli (1 bundle)
- Garlic (2 cloves)
- Eggs and egg whites (2 large, 2 whites)
- Shredded mozzarella cheese (fat-free; ¾ cup)
- Goat cheese (1 tbsp.)
- Kosher salt and ground pepper
- Miso (optional; 1 tbsp.)

How it's made:
To Make the Crust
Heat the oven to 400°F. While the oven preheats, peel your potatoes and be sure to slice them as thinly as possible.

In a glass dish, spread the potatoes in an oval pattern. Lay them well on top of each other so that when they bake and the pieces shrink up, there will be no empty spaces. You might not have to use all the sweet potato you have prepared.

To Make the Quiche

1. Start by baking the crust you made for 15 minutes at 375°F.

2. While that is cooking, chop all of your veggies. Heat up the onion and cook until it's transparent.
3. Next, add the broccoli and kale; cook until they are bright green in color and tender when forked. Add the moisture that has cooked out of the vegetables, which you would have set aside earlier.
4. Lastly, add the garlic and cook until it's light brown
5. Whisk the wet ingredients, eggs, miso and cheeses. Make sure you crumble the goat cheese and stir it in gradually. It will require a few turns of the wrist because of its thickness. Stir the veggies and the eggs together thoroughly.
6. Pour the entire mixture into your potato crust and bake it in the oven for 30 minutes, or until the eggs are formed like a quiche. Serve hot and enjoy.

Asparagus/Eggs Benedict

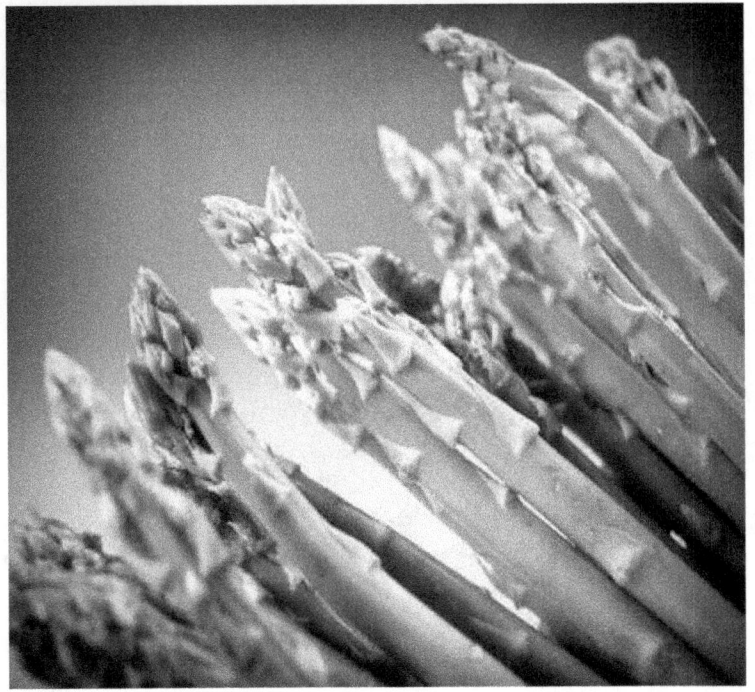

Total Prep & Cooking Time: 35 Minutes
Yields: 4 Servings

What's in it:

- Asparagus stalks (12 ounces)
- Eggs (4 large)
- Apple cider vinegar (2 tsp.)
- Chives for garnish

To Make the Hollandaise Sauce:

- Egg yolks (2 large)

- Ghee (¼ cup)
- Fresh lemon juice (2 tsp.)
- Paprika (¼ tsp.)
- Sea salt (¼ tsp.)

How it's made:

1. Crack open and separate your eggs in a large bowl.
2. Cut off the bottom parts of the asparagus that are rough and not edible. Then, proceed to cut them lengthwise and put them in a large pot. Bring them to a boil and leave them in the water for at least 5 minutes. They should be tender when you stick a fork through.
3. Take the asparagus out of the water with a slotted spoon and add the apple cider vinegar .Turn the heat down to a steady, low simmer.
4. Be careful when adding the eggs so as not to break the yolk. If you have poached egg molds, use those to help it keep its shape.
5. Put a lid on the pan, take it out of the heat, and then continue cooking for 7 to 10 minutes or until you see the yolk of the egg is cooked yet still soft.
6. Drain the eggs on wax paper or paper towels.

How to Make the Sauce

1. Start by adding a bit of boiling water to your blender. Cover the blender with the lid and let stand for at least 12 minutes.
2. Add your egg yolks, lemon juice, salt, and paprika.

3. On a low setting, through the top of the blender, slowly add in your hot butter.
4. Continue to blend for 40 seconds until the sauce has formed and the butter is well-mixed. As it cools, the hollandaise sauce will get thicker.
5. To serve, place each egg over the asparagus spread out on a platter or plate, then put your hollandaise sauce and chopped chives on top.

Bacon & Yam Hash with Celery Root

Total Prep & Cooking Time: 35 Minutes
Yields: 6 Servings

What's in it:

- Bacon, diced (6 to 7 pieces)
- Yam (1 large, cut in ½-inch cubes)
- Celery root, peeled (1, cut in ½-inch cubes)
- Ghee (1-2 tbsp.)
- Onion, diced (1/2 large)
- Garlic, minced (4 cloves)
- Smoked paprika (1 tsp.)
- Sea salt and pepper to taste
- Fresh parsley, minced (1-2 tbsp.)

How it's made:

1. Find a pot that is big enough to hold your yam with plenty of space to spare. Add a pinch of salt to an adequate amount of water for flavor. Add in the yams when the water has reached boiling point.
2. Put the lid on the pot and cook the yams for at least 15 minutes or until your yams are fork tender. Once cooked, drain the yams and be sure to remove as much of the liquid as you can.
3. In a large skillet or sauté pan, fry your bacon pieces until they are crispy but not burnt. Use a spoon with holes to take the bacon out of the pan and place it on a paper towel to remove any of the excess oil.

4. In the same skillet where you cooked the bacon, add your onions and cook them for approximately 5 minutes until they become see-through.
5. Add the celery root and cook it until it's fork tender. You will notice that the celery root will soak up all of the bacon grease in the pan so you will need to add more ghee to keep the hash from burning and/or sticking. Once the celery root is tender, combine the yams and garlic and continue to cook until they turn slightly brown.
6. Be sure to season the hash with salt and pepper generously; slowly and gently mix in the smoked paprika and bacon.
7. Garnish with fresh parsley and enjoy!

Baked Egg and Avocado

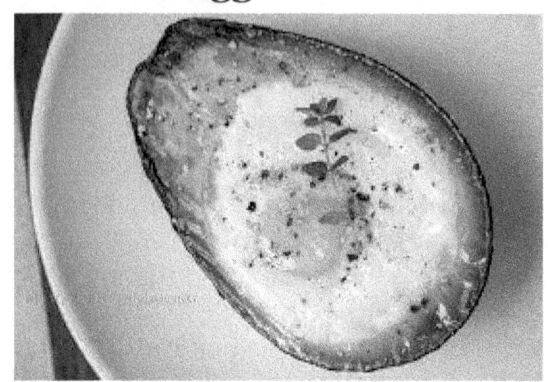

Total Prep & Cooking Time: 20 Minutes
Yields: 2 Servings

What's in it:

- Eggs (2 large)
- Avocado (1 large)
- Lemon (1/2, squeezed)
- Sea salt and pepper to taste

How it's made:

1. Prepare by getting the oven temperature up to 425°F.
2. Use an ice cream scoop (if you have it) to carve out the entire inside of the avocado; be sure to leave at least a ½-inch rim.
3. Crack open the egg directly on top of the avocado once you have loosened it from the shell. Don't worry about any excess running off; it happens.
4. Add the squeezed lemon juice, salt, and pepper to both avocado halves.

5. Bake each half in the oven for at least 15 minutes or until you can see the yolks set.

Breakfast Pizza Quiche Style

Total Prep & Cooking Time: 35 Minutes
Yields: 4 Servings

What's in it:

- Ghee, melted (1 tsp.)
- Eggs(8 large)
- Coconut milk (1/4 cup)
- Garlic powder (1/2 tsp.)
- Salt (to your taste)
- Black pepper (1/2 tsp.)
- Dried oregano (1/4 tsp.)
- Mushrooms, sliced (1 1/2 cups)
- Roasted red pepper, sliced (1/2 cup)
- Pepperoni, quartered (3 ounces)
- Onion powder (1/2 tsp.)
- Green onions, chopped(1/4 cup)
- Pizza sauce (2 tbsp.)

How it's made:

1. Bring the oven temperature to 375°F.
2. Grease a 10-inch baking dish. You can line this with parchment paper if you have some on hand; if not, the melted ghee will be fine.
3. Break open all of the eggs in a large bowl and mix in coconut milk. Blend together until they're well-combined.
4. Add the dry seasonings and continue to mix well.

5. After you have combined the ingredients, continue adding the veggies with the pepperoni and green onions. Whisk all the ingredients until they're thoroughly mixed.
6. Add mixture into the pan along with the pizza sauce and pepperoni.
7. Bake in the oven on 375°F for at least 25 minutes. Let stand for at least 10 minutes before you cut and serve.

Sweet Potato Boat

Total Prep & Cooking Time: 15 Minutes
Yields: 4 Servings

What's in it:

- Sweet potatoes (4)
- Bacon (2 pieces)
- Ground beef(1 pound)
- Sea salt (½ tsp.)
- Olive oil (2 tsp.)
- Ghee(½ tsp.)
- Cinnamon (½ tsp.)
- Onion powder (½ tsp.)
- Paprika (½ tsp.)
- Chopped scallions (2 tsp.)

How it's made:

1. Clean the potatoes in warm water and bake in the oven at 400°F until fork tender.
2. Cook the bacon. In a large skillet, with ¼ teaspoon of sea salt, brown the ground beef and add the olive oil.
3. Combine all of the dry spices in a bowl and mix well. While waiting for the ground beef to brown, cut up the scallions.
4. When the sweet potatoes are cooked, slice them in half but do not cut all the way.
5. Add a small amount of the ghee to the top of the sweet potato and sprinkle the ¼ teaspoon

of sea salt and the rest of the seasonings you mixed earlier for flavor.
6. Top each sweet potato with the ground beef and scallions and bake in the oven for 5-10 minutes.

Avocado Toast

Total Prep & Cooking Time: 10 Minutes
Yields: 1 Serving

What's in it:

- Sweet potato (1 large)
- Avocado (1)
- Olive oil (1-2 tbsp.)
- Lime wedges
- Sesame seeds
- Sliced green onions
- Garlic powder, to taste
- Salt and pepper, to taste

How it's made:

1. Dice the sweet potato into large chunks and coat with the olive oil, garlic, and salt and pepper to your desired taste.
2. In a large skillet and using a medium to high heat setting, cook the potato until you can stick a fork all the way through and it's completely browned on the outside. It will take about 10 minutes for each side.
3. Slice the avocado and lay it across the top of the sweet potatoes.
4. Garnish the dish with sesame seeds, green onions, salt, pepper, crushed red pepper, and lime juice.

Mango wrapped in Prosciutto

Total Prep & Cooking Time: 10 Minutes
Yields: 1 Serving

What's in it:

- Mango (1 large)
- Wholefood-compliant prosciutto (1 package)
- Arugula (2 bunches)

How it's made:

1. First, peel the mango and cut it into long, thick spear-like slices.
2. Next, take each spear of mango and simply wrap the prosciutto around it. Serve over your favorite bed of quinoa or lettuce.

Sausage Balls

Total Prep & Cooking Time: 30 Minutes
Yields: 2 Servings

What's in it:

- Sweet potato (1 large)
- Dijon mustard (organic, 1 tbsp.)
- Coconut flour (1/3 cup)
- Organic butter (2 tbsp.)
- Veggie trio of onion, carrot ,and celery (chopped, 2 tbsp.)
- Italian seasoning (2 tsp.)
- Eggs (2 large)
- Sea salt and pepper, to taste
- Pork sausage or chorizo (1 pound)

How it's made:

1. Begin by bringing the oven temperature to 350°F.
2. Place the sweet potato in the microwave-safe dish and add in a dash of water (about half an inch or so is fine).Cover the dish with a paper towel if it does not have a lid. Microwave for 6 minutes on high heat until its fork tender .Let it sit and cool off before you peel and dice it.
3. While the potato is cooking, in a separate skillet, cook the sausage until it's halfway done. Add the seasonings and chopped veggies, along with the mustard and Italian seasoning. Cook

the sausage until brown and drain the excess oil on a paper towel.
4. When cooked, add the potato in a mixing bowl and mash thoroughly. Combine with the remaining ingredients and continue stirring.
5. Next, add the eggs so they don't scramble from the hot sausage and then mix until well-blended.
6. Using an ice cream scooper, scoop out at least 2 teaspoons of the potato. Roll it into a ball then place on a lined baking sheet.
7. Cook for 30-35 minutes or until cooked. Let it sit for 15 minutes before serving.

Guacamole & Bacon Sandwich

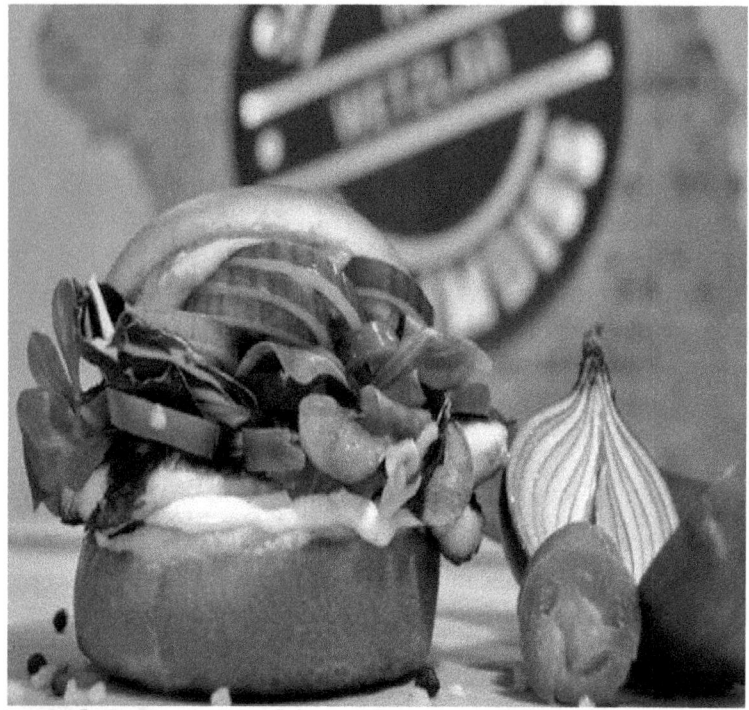

Total Prep & Cooking Time: 10 Minutes
Yields: 1 Serving

What's in it:

- Nitrate-free bacon (4 strips of thick cuts)
- Hass avocado (1 medium)
- Lime (1)
- Kosher salt (as desired)

How it's made:

1. Wrap the slices of bacon in thick sheets of paper towels and place them on a microwave-

safe dish; microwave until crispy (microwave settings will vary).
2. Take half of the avocado flesh and mash it. Then, take the other half and cut it into cubes. Mix both of the halves in a bowl together. You should have a nice creamy, chunky mixture.
3. Season with the lime juice and kosher salt and enjoy!

Sweet Potato & Zucchini Cakes

Total Prep & Cooking Time: 30 Minutes
Yields: 4 Servings

What's in it:

- Shredded zucchini(1 cup)
- Shredded sweet potato (1 cup)
- Egg, beaten (1)
- Coconut flour (1 tbsp.)
- Garlic powder (1/2 tsp.)
- Ground cumin (1/4 tsp.)
- Dried parsley (1/2 tsp.)
- Salt and pepper (to taste)
- Ghee (1 tbsp.)
- EV olive oil (1 tbsp.)

How it's made:

1. In a medium bowl, combine zucchini, sweet potato, and egg.
2. In another mixing bowl, combine the dry spices with the coconut flour. Add the dry seasonings and ingredients to the mixture and stir well.
3. Using a medium heat setting, cook the ghee and olive. Separate the mixture into four equal parts and add to the pan. Press down with a fork until you get ½-inch thick patties.
4. Continue to cook on medium heat until the patties are crispy and golden brown; once they're brown on one side, flip carefully and cook the other side.

5. Drain on a paper towel or rack .Sprinkle with the kosher salt while they're still hot. Enjoy!

Simple Granola Bars

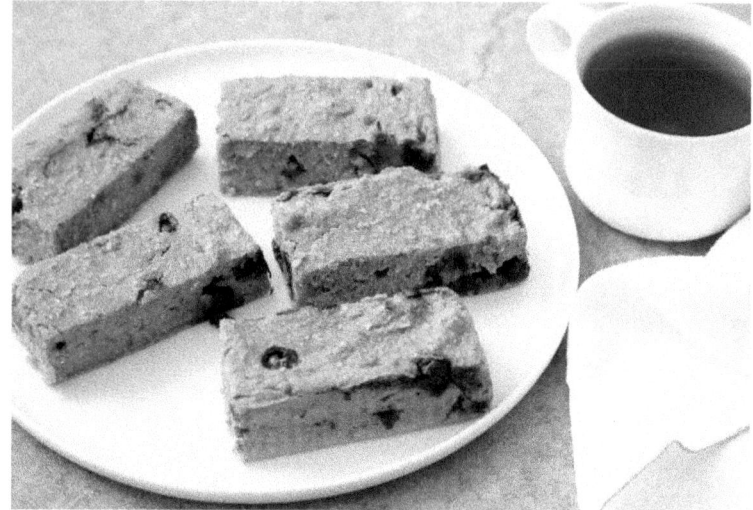

Total Prep & Cooking Time: 10 Minutes
Yields: 2 Servings

What's in it:

- Pitted dates (1 cup)
- Walnuts or Brazil nuts (2 cups)
- Desiccated coconut (2 cups)
- Cranberries, dried (¾ cup)
- Water (3 tbsp.)

How it's made:

1. Begin by lightly toasting the walnuts in a heated stove set at 170°F. After they cool off, add them to your mixer with the coconut, date, and cranberries and mix until it all becomes crumbled.

2. Slowly add the water one tablespoon at a time until the crumbled texture turns sticky and it appears to hold together on its own.
3. Place a layer of non-stick cling wrap to the bottom of a pan and place your mixture in the top middle. Make sure to press down firmly.
4. Next, get a square baking dish, line it up with cling film and pour the mixture in. Press down firmly to ensure the mixture sticks well together.
5. Pop in the fridge for a couple of hours, then cut into bars and sprinkle with some more desiccated coconut.

Breakfast Burrito

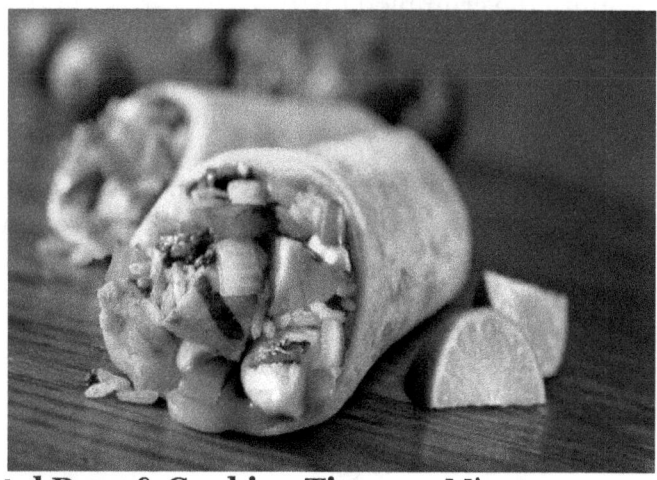

Total Prep & Cooking Time: 10 Minutes
Yields: 1 Serving

What's in it:

- Sliced ham
- Egg whites (2)
- Chopped veggies (1/4 cup)
- Optional: salsa, guacamole, cilantro

How it's made:

1. In a large saucepan, cook the veggies in a small bit of ghee over medium-high heat.
2. Combine the eggs and veggie mix in a small bowl and whisk.
3. Scramble the mixture as you would normally scramble eggs and then remove from the pan when cooked.

4. Add the ham around the pan and eggs and put it back on the heat. You can add salsa, or guacamole, on top for extra flavor.

Lunch Recipes

Try these delicious lunch recipes to keep building your relationship with food and to maintain the integrity of your whole food lifestyle. Enjoy!

Sweet Potato Fries with Guacamole

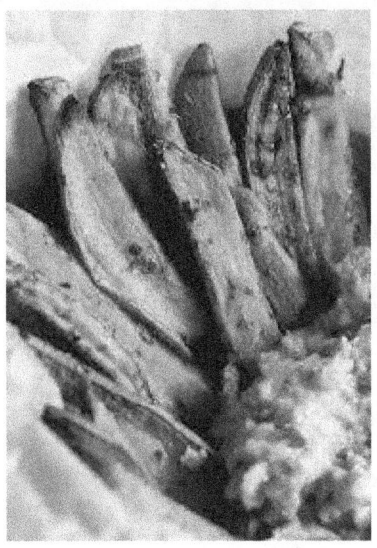

Total Prep & Cooking Time: 60 Minutes
Yields: 4 Servings

What's in it:

- Sweet potatoes cut in wedges (3 medium)
- Avocado oil (5 tbsp.)
- Smoked paprika (1 tbsp.)
- Cinnamon (1 tsp.)
- Cayenne pepper powder (1/4 tsp.)
- Nutmeg (1/4 tsp.)
- Ground ginger (1/4 tsp.)
- Cracked black pepper and salt, to taste (1 tsp.)
- Avocados (3 mashed)
- Onion (1 small, diced into small cubes)

- Tomatoes (2, cut)
- Garlic (2 cloves, minced)
- Lime juice (1 lime)
- Salt and pepper (as desired)

How it's made:

1. Begin by preheating the oven to 400°F.

2. Combine all of the ingredients besides the guacamole ingredients in a large bowl.

3. Take some parchment or wax paper and put it in the bottom of the pan. Spread the sweet potatoes in one layer on the bottom.

4. Bake in the oven on 400°F for about 40 minutes or until you see the potatoes are crispy. Check every 15 minutes as oven temperatures may vary.

Ground Turkey Nachos

Total Prep & Cooking Time: 20 Minutes
Yields: 2 Servings

What's in it:

- Taco shells (8 hard)
- Canola oil (1 tbsp.)
- Ground turkey (1 pound)
- Homemade taco seasoning mix (2 tbsp.)
- Tomatoes (diced)
- Onions (diced)
- Pico de gallo (homemade)
- Sliced avocados
- Cheese, non-dairy
- Fresh cilantro (chopped)

How it's made:

1. Heat the oven to 200°F. Begin by warming up the taco shells on a baking or cookie sheet.

2. Over medium heat, add the turkey and oil in a large skillet and brown; stir the turkey occasionally.

3. Mix the taco seasoning with 1/4 cup of water and add it to the turkey. Keep cooking until all of the liquid is gone from the turkey meat.

4. Fill your taco shells like you see them do at taco bars and enjoy.

Fiesta Chicken Salad

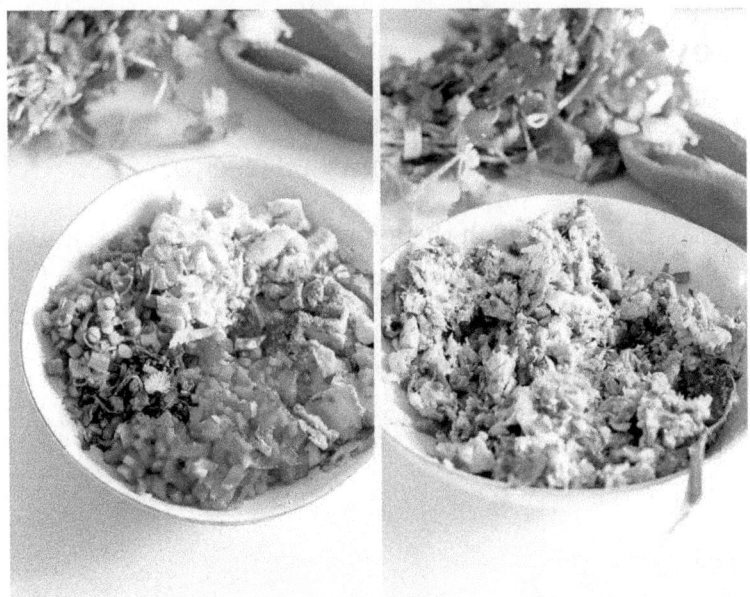

Total Prep & Cooking Time: 5 Minutes
Yields: 4 Servings

What's in it:

- Avocado (1)
- Chicken, cooked and shredded (2 cups)
- Red bell pepper (1/2, finely diced)
- Fresh cilantro (1/4 cup, chopped)
- Scallions (2, thinly sliced)
- Lime juice (1 lime)
- Cumin (1/4 tsp.)
- Smoked paprika (1/4 tsp.)
- Cayenne pepper (dash)

- Salt and pepper (as desired)

How it's made:

1. Prepare and cook the chicken beforehand or use leftovers from a previous recipe.

2. Mix and mash the avocado in a large bowl and then mix in the rest of the ingredients. Enjoy!

Turkey Burgers with Jalapeno

Total Prep & Cooking Time: 30 Minutes
Yields: 2 Servings

What's in it:

- Ground turkey (1 pound)
- Jalapeño pepper, minced (1/2 to 3/4)
- Shallot, peeled (1 medium, minced)
- Lime juice and zest (2 tsp. each)
- Chopped cilantro (2 tbsp.)
- Paprika (1 tsp.)
- Cumin (1 tsp.)
- Sea salt (1/2 tsp.)
- Black pepper (1/2 tsp.)
- Guacamole
- Pico de gallo
- Poached egg (optional)

How it's made:

1. Be sure to look for a ground turkey brand that has the consistency of hamburger meat. If what you found has a lot of liquid, drain it really well before cooking.

2. Using your hands, mix together the turkey, spices, herbs, lime zest, and lime juice in a

bowl. Shape the combination into four burger patties.

3. In a skillet, using a heat setting of medium to high, add your olive oil followed by your patties. Cook for about 5 minutes on each side and top with the guacamole and/or the pico de gallo if desired.

Cauliflower Soup with Turkey and Kale

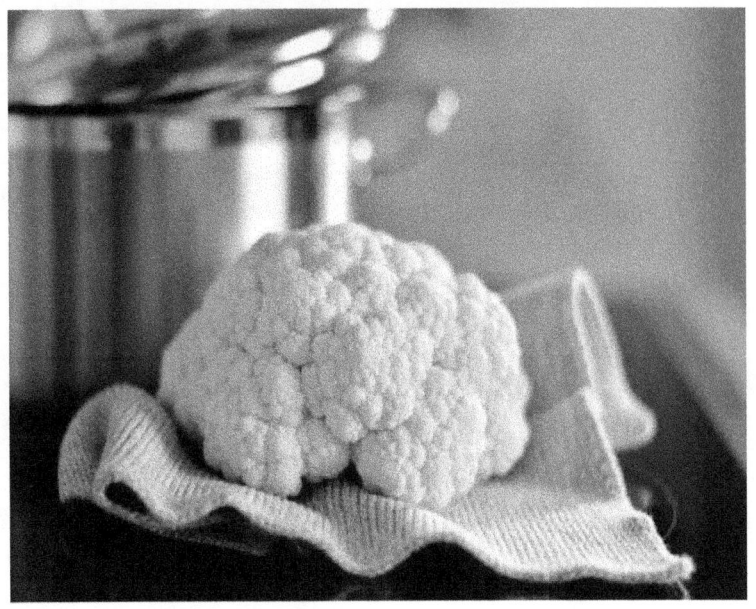

Total Prep & Cooking Time: 45 Minutes
Yields: 4 Servings

What's in it:

- Ground turkey (1 pound)
- Shallots (4, chopped)
- Carrots (3, sliced)
- Bell pepper (1, cut and diced)
- Diced tomatoes (15 oz. can)
- Chicken stock (5 cups)
- Cauliflower (1 ½ cup, minced)
- Kale, leaves only (4 cups, coarsely chopped)
- Coconut oil (2 tbsp.)

- Sea salt and black pepper (as desired)

How it's made:

1. Over medium-high heat, add the coconut oil in a large saucepan.

2. Cook for 1-2 minutes, then add the shallots, carrots, cauliflower, and bell pepper.

3. Cook until the vegetables are tender, typically between 8 and 10 minutes; be sure to stir frequently.

4. Cook for 10 minutes or so, then add your turkey meat and cook until it's completely well done, which takes about 6 to 8 minutes.

5. Pour in the chicken stock, add the tomatoes, and season with pepper and salt as you normally would.

6. Bring it all to a boil, stirring once; turn the heat to simmer and cover. Cook for an additional 15 minutes while covered. Serve and enjoy hot!

Asparagus Bundles with Salmon

Total Prep & Cooking Time: 25 Minutes
Yields: 4 Servings

What's in it:

- Smoked salmon (4 oz.)
- Asparagus spears (1 pound)
- Olive oil (1 tbsp.)
- Salt (1/4 tsp.)
- Paprika (1/8 tsp.)
- Cayenne pepper (1 pinch)
- Garlic powder (1/8 tsp.)
- Red bell pepper (1 medium)

How it's made:

1. Begin by heating your oven to 425°F. Prepare your pan or baking sheet with foil for later use.

2. Cut off the ends of the asparagus spears. Lightly coat them with the oil, salt, garlic powder, paprika, and cayenne pepper. Place the asparagus in your pan or baking sheet.

3. Cut the bell pepper in half, remove the seeds inside, and place it on the baking sheet alongside the asparagus.

4. Cook in the preheated oven for about 10 minutes; mix on occasion, and continue cooking for about 8-10 minutes. Take the pan out of the oven and let it cool off for a few minutes.

5. Cut the bell pepper into bite-sized chunks and bundle the asparagus, about 4-5 spears in each, and add a few slices of the bell pepper slices into each bundle. Turn the oven setting to broil.

6. Take a piece of salmon and wrap each asparagus bundle with it. Place all the bundles back on the baking sheet and broil in the oven for about 3 minutes. Enjoy!

Tuna Salad with Avocado

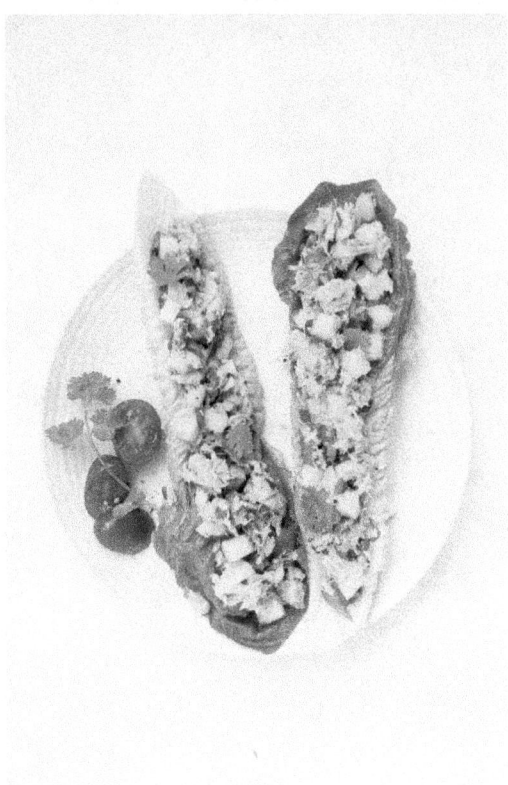

Total Prep & Cooking Time: 10 Minutes
Yields: 6 Servings

What's in it:

- Tuna in oil (3 15-oz. cans)
- English cucumber (1, sliced)
- Avocados (2 large or 3 medium)
- Red onion (1 small/medium, thinly sliced)
- Cilantro (1/4 cup)
- EV olive oil (2 tbsp.)

- Lemon juice (2 tbsp.)
- Black pepper (1/8 tsp.)
- Sea salt (1 tsp.)

How it's made:

1. Grab a large bowl, add the cucumber, sliced avocado, sliced red onion, flaked and drained tuna, and cilantro.
2. Sprinkle the salad ingredients with lemon juice and olive oil, along with the black pepper and salt to taste; mix and serve!

Poached Salmon with Carrots

Total Prep & Cooking Time: 30 Minutes
Yields: 4 Servings

What's in it:

- Carrots (about 6 oz.)
- Vegetable broth(1 cup, no salt)
- Fresh flat-leaf parsley, chopped(1 tbsp.)
- Salmon fillet with skin (1 piece,5 oz.)
- Sea salt (pinch)

How it's made:

1. In a deep skillet, add the carrots and broth. Sprinkle the parsley on top and bring everything to a slow boil.
2. Let cook for 5 minutes then reduce the heat and cover. Continue to cook for an additional 5 minutes.
3. Take the lid off and push the carrots to the entire outside rim of the pan. Add the salmon, skin-side down, directly in the middle of the pan; season with the sea salt.
4. Return the lid and continue to cook and simmer until the salmon is cooked all the way through and is light pink in color at the center. The carrots should be extremely tender after cooking for at least 12 minutes more.
5. Keep the salmon in the fridge for up to 2 days. If you plan on eating it much later, freeze the part you want to save.

Fresh Seafood Salad

Total Prep & Cooking Time: 60 Minutes
Yields: 8 Servings

What's in it:

- EV olive oil, divided (4 tbsp.)
- Fresh lime juice (2 tbsp.)
- Grated lime peels (2 tbsp.)
- Honey (1 1/2 tbsp.)
- Salt (1/2 tsp.)
- Ground chipotle pepper (1/4 tsp.)
- Skinless salmon fillet (1 ½ pound, diced into 1 1/4-inch pieces)
- Sea scallops (18 large)
- Mussels, scrubbed (2 dozen, de-bearded)
- Manila clams (2 dozen, scrubbed)

How it's made:

1. Combine 2 tbsp. of the oil and the next five ingredients into a bowl size of your choice. Place the salmon and scallops on opposite sides of a glass baking dish. No overlapping.
2. Cover the seafood with the marinade and make sure to completely coat it without letting the fish touch. Allow it to marinade on the counter for 1 hour, flipping the meat mid-way through. Drain each by itself and keep the leftover marinade separate.
3. Heat the rest of the olive oil on medium heat. Season the fish with salt and pepper. Place the

salmon in the skillet and cook until it has a light pink center, typically about 3 minutes.
4. Transfer the salmon to the serving platter. Next, cook the scallops for about 1 1/2 minutes per side.
5. Add the scallops with the salmon on the platter and cover with the marinade. Add the mussels and clams. Cook until they are completely open and you can see inside the shell. This typically takes about 3 minutes. Throw out any shellfish that do not open.
6. Add the mussels and clams to the dish of salmon and scallops and allow it to reach room temperature .Season the seafood with some cilantro dressing.

Apple & Ginger Smoothie

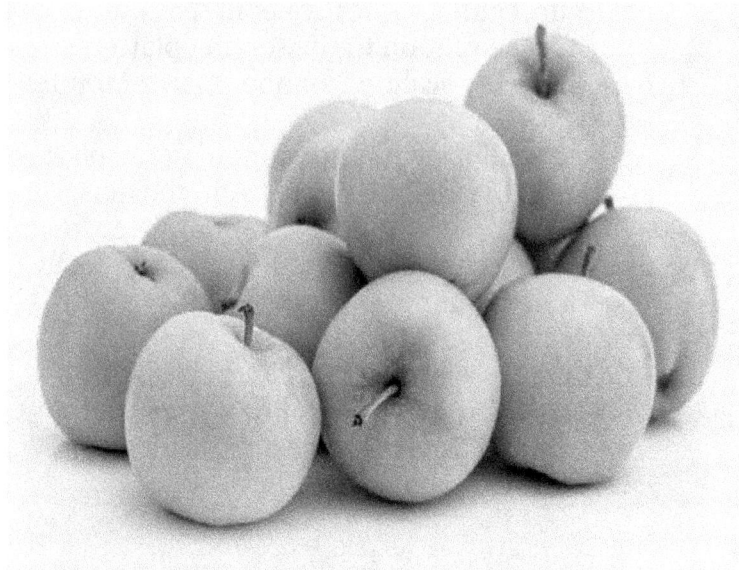

Total Prep & Cooking Time: 5 Minutes
Yields: 2 Servings

What's in it:

- Water (1 cup)
- Oranges (2)
- Apple (1)
- Spinach (1 cup)
- Banana (1, peeled)
- Lemon (1, peeled)
- Strawberries (8, frozen)
- Fresh ginger (2 tsp.)
- Ice (1 cup)

How it's made:

1. Simply add all the above ingredients into your favorite blender, mix well, pour into a glass, and enjoy!

Shredded Pork and Warm Potato Salad

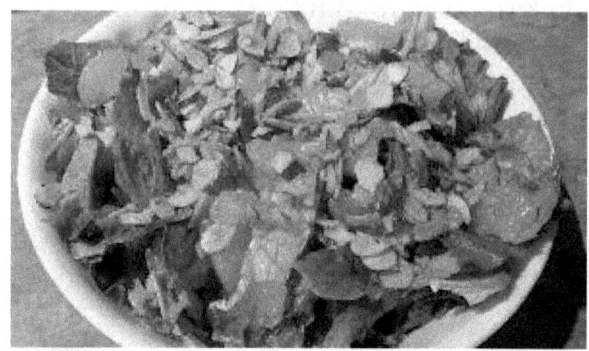

Total Prep & Cooking Time: 20 minutes
Yields: 3 Servings

What's in it:

- EV olive oil (2 tbsp.)
- Lemon (½, juiced)
- Paprika (¼ tsp.)
- Salt and pepper
- Baked potatoes (3 medium)
- Slow-cooker pork (9 oz.; this can be taken from leftovers)
- Cucumber, seedless (1 large; cut in 1-inch pieces)
- Avocado (½ large)
- Fresh parsley (3 tbsp.)

How it's made:

1. In a large mixing bowl, toss together all of the dry ingredients and divide it into four containers; these will make four servings for the weeks' lunch or snacks.

2. In another mixing bowl, combine the lemon juice, olive oil, and paprika. Using salt and pepper, season the mixture to taste.
3. Lastly, add the potatoes along with the pork and cover completely, turning occasionally to make sure it's completely covered.
4. When reheating, do so for only 90 seconds.

Pita Pocket with Avocado, Lettuce, and Tomato

Total Prep & Cooking Time: 10 Minutes
Yields: 4 Servings

What's in it:

- Avocado (1 large)
- Red wine vinegar (1 tbsp.)
- Pinch fine sea salt
- Pinch ground black pepper
- Grain pita pockets (2 whole)
- Butter lettuce leaves (4)
- Basil (1/4 cup)
- Tomatoes (2 medium, cut into 4 slices)

How it's made:

1. Combine and mash the avocado with vinegar, salt, and pepper until everything is smooth in texture.
2. Cut the pita pockets in half and fill them with lettuce leaves and basil.
3. Evenly split up the avocado mixture between pita pockets; be sure to coat the lettuce leaves. Add 2 tomato slices to each pocket. Serve and enjoy!

Bean Salad with Green Onion & Carrots

Total Prep & Cooking Time: 20 Minutes
Yields: 4 Servings

What's in it:

- Cider vinegar or rice vinegar (3 tbsp.)
- Low-sodium tamari (1 tbsp.)
- Mustard, preferably German (1 tsp.)
- Tahini (1 tbsp.)
- No-salt chickpeas (2 1/2 cups)
- Thinly sliced green onions (1/2 cup)
- Grated carrots (1/2 cup)
- Fresh flat-leaf parsley (1/2 bunch, chopped)

How it's made:

1. Mix together your vinegar, mustard, tahini, and at least 3 tbsp. of the water in a bowl.
2. Put in the beans, carrots, and green onions next, then toss in the parsley. Mix all of that together and leave it to set on the counter at room temperature for about 15 minutes.
3. Plate and serve.

Veggie Pizza with Hummus

Total Prep & Cooking Time: 20 Minutes
Yields: 4 Servings

What's in it:

- Vegetable broth, low-sodium (1/2 cup)
- Balsamic vinegar (3 tbsp.)
- Roasted red pepper hummus (1 1/2 cup, divided)
- Portobello mushroom caps (1 1/2 cup)
- Yellow squash (1; sliced lengthwise into 1/3-inch planks)
- Tortillas (4 whole)
- Baby spinach, lightly steamed (8 oz.)
- Chopped fresh basil (1/4 cup)
- Pine nuts (1/4 cup)
- Ground black pepper (to taste)
- Zucchini (1; sliced lengthwise and cut into 1/3-inch pieces)

How it's made:

1. Combine the broth, balsamic vinegar, and hummus.
2. Next, add the mushrooms and coat evenly. Take a slotted spoon and remove it from the bowl; add the yellow squash and zucchini and coat as well.
3. Add the mushrooms back in; let the vegetables sit to marinade for about 8 minutes.

4. Preheat your grill pan on medium heat and grill the vegetables until they're tender and crispy, about 4 minutes on each side. Put them to the side.
5. Set the temperature on your oven to 375°F. Put tortillas on a pan or baking sheet and spread each with the leftover hummus. Once finished, you can add the spinach, basil, and grilled vegetables on top.
6. Continue to cook in the oven until the corners of the tortillas are brown and crisp and the pine nuts are golden brown; this should all take about 15 minutes.
7. Cut and enjoy.

Sweet Greens Smoothie

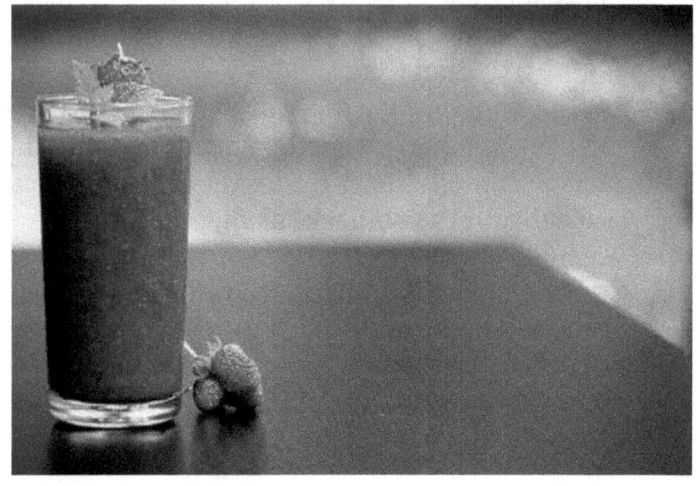

Total Prep & Cooking Time: 5 Minutes
Yields: 2 Servings

What's in it:

- Water (1 cup)
- Spinach (1 cup)
- Banana (2)
- Grapes (2 cups)
- Kale (1 piece, ribbed)
- Parsley (2 sprigs)
- Cucumber (⅓)
- Celery (⅓)
- Flaxseed oil (optional; 1 tbsp.)

How it's made:

1. Combine all the ingredients in a blender and blend until they're thoroughly combined.

2. Serve cold.

Dinner Recipes

Try these delicious dinner recipes to keep building your relationship with food and to maintain the integrity of your whole food lifestyle. Enjoy!

Veggie Burgers with Plantains and Black Beans

Total Prep & Cooking Time: 25 Minutes
Yields: 4 Servings

What's in it:

- Plantain (1 ripe; large, blackened, and peeled)
- Black beans (1 can; drained and rinsed)
- Hemp seeds (1/4 cup)
- Tahini (1 1/2 tbsp.)
- Lime juice (1 tbsp.)
- Red onion (1/4 cup, chopped)
- Finely chopped cilantro (2 tbsp.)
- Oat flour (1-2 tbsp.)
- Salt (pinch)
- Chipotle powder (1/2 tsp.)
- Optional toppers: avocado, onion, tomato
- Optional condiments: home-made salsa, homemade mayo

How it's made:

1. Start by slicing the plantains thinly .In a skillet over high heat, add 1 tsp. of oil. Add the plantains to the hot pan and cook for about 3 minutes on each side.

2. The plantains are going to turn a brownish color, which is fine. Be sure to add a touch of water if the pan seems to be getting too dry. Take the plantains out of the pan; set aside 1 cup and put it in the bowl.

3. Add the bean, flour, chipotle powder, onion, and salt. Then, add the seeds, tahini, cilantro, and lime. Mash the beans until they have completely split apart; use a masher or a fork.

4. Add another teaspoon of oil to a medium-high heat skillet. Create patties and keep putting them in the hot skillet until the liquid has evaporated.

5. Cook for about 1-3 minutes on each side. Simply assemble the burgers to your preference.

Soba Noodle Salad with Brussels Sprouts

Total Prep & Cooking Time: 20 Minutes
Yields: 4 Servings

What's in it:

- Brussels sprouts (8 large)
- Garlic (1 clove)
- Tuscan kale (5 oz.; you can also use a 5-oz. box of baby kale)
- Soba noodles (8 oz.)
- Soy sauce (1 tsp.)
- Brown rice wine vinegar (1 tbsp.)
- Sesame seeds, toasted (1 tbsp.)
- Red chili flakes (2 pinches)
- Sesame oil, divided (8 tsp.)
- Chives (1/2 cup)
- Sea salt

How it's made:

1. Boil a big pot of water that has sea salt added. Cook the soba noodles as indicated by the bundle instructions. Strain, then toss with 3 tsp. of the sesame oil.

2. As you wait for the noodles to cook, set up the veggies. Clean the kale under running water

and dry. If you've chosen Tuscan kale, strip the stems of their leaves. Bunch them up in a neat stack and cut them into thin strips. Place the strips in a huge bowl.

3. If you are using baby kale, put the cleaned and dried leaves into the bowl. Include 1/4 tsp. sea salt and 2 tsp. of the sesame oil and rub these into the leaves with your hands until they have begun to wilt; make sure they are completely coated.

4. Pound the garlic into a paste-like texture, with salt added. Mix in the rice vinegar. Add the rest of the sesame oil and soy sauce and stir until you have a smooth dressing. Pour over the kale and Brussels sprouts, tossing them well to coat.

5. Next, toss the cooked noodles, sesame seeds, and red chili pieces. Top with chives or scallions and serve chilled or at room temperature.

Quinoa Bowl

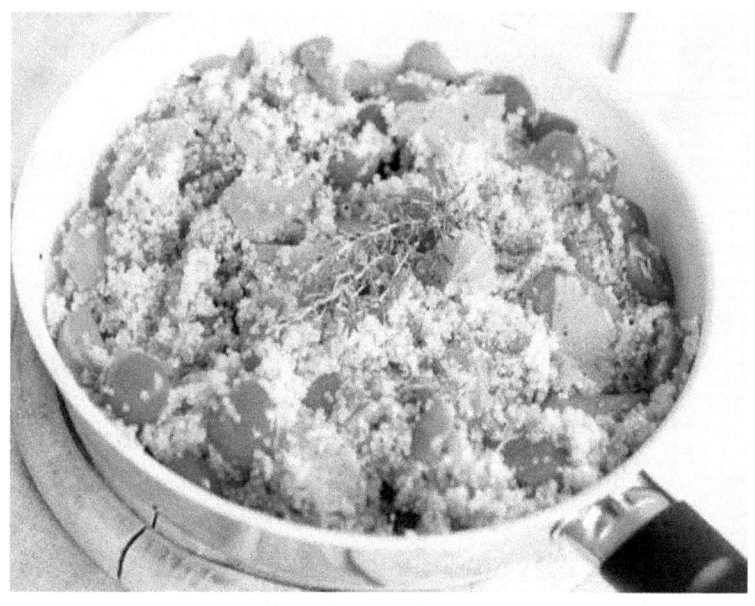

Total Prep & Cooking Time: 10 Minutes
Yields: 1 Serving

What's in it:

- Kale or greens of choice (1 cup)
- Cooked quinoa (1/2 cup)
- Cooked lentils or beans of choice (1/2 cup)
- Brussels sprouts, roasted (1/2 cup)
- Butternut squash, roasted (1/2 cup)
- Avocado (1)
- Tahini dressing

For the Salad Dressing:

- Tahini (1 tbsp.)
- Lemon juice (1 tsp.)
- Wheat-free tamari (1/2 tsp.)
- Water, as needed (1/2 tsp.)

How it's made:

1. Start by arranging your greens at the bottom of a glass baking dish, then put the other ingredients in layers on top.

2. Blend the dressing ingredients together in a bowl, then simply top the bowl with the dressing.

Slow Cooker Chicken with Salsa

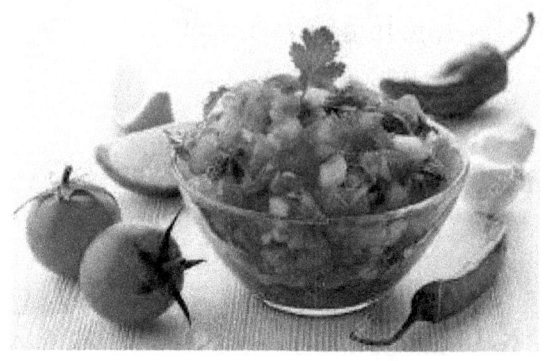

Total Prep & Cooking Time: 6-8 Hours (advanced preparation)
Yields: 3 Servings

What's in it:

- Boneless, skinless chicken breasts (1 lb.; about 2)
- Salsa (1 1/2 cups; your favorite type)

How it's made:

1. Add the whole uncooked chicken breasts to your slow cooker and cover them with the salsa. Place the lid on the slow cooker and cook on high for about 4 hours. Alternatively, you can place it on low for 6-8 hours to get the same desired results.

2. Use the remaining salsa and juice to cover the chicken when done. Serve hot or store in the

fridge in an airtight bowl or container; good for at least 5 days.

BBQ Lentil Burgers with Chickpea French Fries

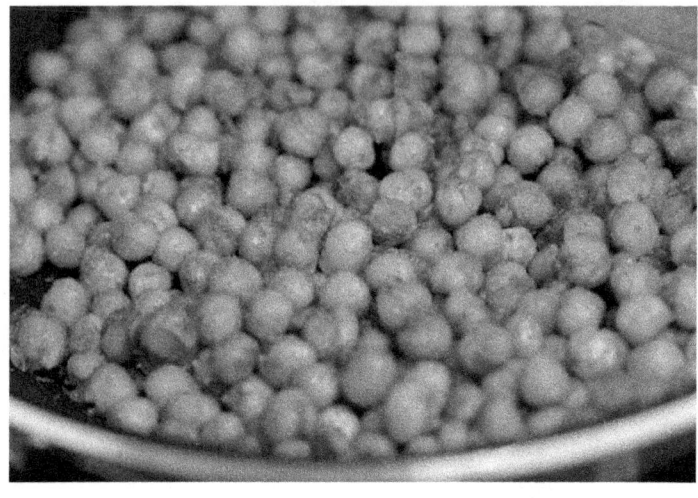

Total Prep & Cooking Time: 25 Minutes
Yields: 4 Servings

What's in it:

- Brown lentils (1½ cups)
- Water (4½ cups)
- Olive oil (1 tbsp.)
- Onion, chopped (¾ cup)
- Shitake mushroom (6 oz.)
- Sun-dried tomatoes (½ cup)
- Garlic, minced (3 cloves)
- Smoked paprika (½ tsp.)
- Chili powder (1 tsp.)
- Thyme (½ tsp.)

- Oregano
- Walnuts, raw (¾ cup)
- Rolled oats (½ cup)
- Salt (½ tsp.)
- Breadcrumbs (½ cup)
- Black pepper

Prepare the Barbecue Sauce:

- Tomato paste (¼ cup)
- Maple syrup (2 tbsp.)
- Molasses (blackstrap; ½ tbsp.)
- Tamari (2 tbsp.)
- Tamarind concentrate (1½ tbsp.)
- Apple cider vinegar (1½ tbsp.)
- Chili powder (½ tsp.)
- Ground coriander (½ tsp.)
- Garlic, minced (1 clove)
- Ginger powder (½ tsp.)
- Black pepper

Prepare the Fries:

- Chickpea flour (2 cups)
- Water (4 cups)
- Salt (1½ tsp.)
- Cumin (1 tsp.)
- Garlic, chopped (1 clove)
- Parsley, chopped (½ cup)

- Olive oil

How it's made:

1. Start by making the barbecue sauce. Mix all the ingredients well, with the exception of the pepper. Taste the seasoning and add extra pepper if desired. Put in a closed container and refrigerate for up to 4 days.

2. To make the burgers, start by sorting and picking your beans to remove any that are bad. Run the good beans under extremely cold water, then put them in a medium- to large-sized pot and boil. Reduce the heat and simmer the beans for at least 20 minutes until they are completely fork tender and falling apart. Take them off the stove, drain, and put to the side for later use.

3. Heat up the oil in a large skillet. Make sure the heat is on at least medium-high. Put in the onion and season with the salt and pepper; cook for at least 5 minutes .Next, add your mushrooms and simmer for 5 minutes. Mushrooms release liquid; when they are no longer doing so, they are done.

4. Delicious sun-dried tomatoes and garlic go in next. Simmer for another minute or two until you can smell the garlic in the air. Add a few

drops of the broth to keep them from sticking to the pan.

5. Add in all of your dry ingredients along with the beans and mix them all together to make sure they are evenly distributed. Take them off the heat.

6. Make sure the oven's temperature has been preheated to 350°F. Put in the walnuts and oats in a blender and add a ½ tsp. of salt. Set the blender on pulse; mix and blend until both the oats and nuts are in a powder form.

7. Add your bean mixture and give it a few more pulses until it turns into a puree. Pour this mixture into a bowl and, with your hands, begin to make your burgers. You should be able to get eight out of this recipe.

8. Put the burgers on a baking sheet and brush it with the tamarind and barbeque sauce. Cook for 15 minutes. Be sure to turn the burgers over and brush the other side. Keep cooking for 10 minutes or until the burger is crispy on the outside. You can serve this on any Wholefood bun of your choice.

9. To make the fries, put the chickpea flour, reserved water, salt, cumin, and garlic into a mixer and blend until smooth.

10. Put all of that mixture into a pot and put it on the stove on medium-high heat; cook while stirring often. It is going to thicken up quickly, so be sure to keep an eye on it. Have your whisk and some water handy to loosen it up.

11. While it is still hot, put the mixture onto a lined baking sheet and smooth it out evenly all over. Put this in the fridge to set for at least an hour.

12. About 10 minutes before you take the mixture out of the fridge, heat up the oven to 375°F. Take the dough out and begin to cut it into strips about three inches long. Brush them with oil as you cut them.

13. Bake for at least 15 minutes. Turn them slowly and continue to brush them with oil as they cook. Cook an additional 12 minutes and serve with the tahini dressing if you like. Enjoy!

Cauliflower Bowl (Spicy)

Total Prep & Cooking Time: 30 Minutes
Yields: 4 Servings

What's in it:

- Cauliflower, chopped into florets (1 head)
- EV olive oil (1 tbsp.)
- Salt and pepper
- Hot sauce (1/3 cup)
- Sriracha (3 tbsp.)
- Ghee (1 tbsp.)
- Coconut milk (3 tbsp.)
- Quinoa, dry (1 cup)
- Water (2 cups)
- Yellow onion, diced (1 medium)
- Kale, steamed or sautéed (1 cup)
- Chickpeas (1 1/2 cups; cooked or canned)
- Avocado, diced (1)
- Chopped parsley to garnish

How it's made:

1. Preheat the broiler to 400°F.

2. Cleave one head of cauliflower into florets and shower with 1 tbsp. of olive oil, salt, and pepper.

3. Spread evenly onto a baking dish or cookie sheet and cook for 30 minutes, tossing them about halfway through the cooking time.

4. Boil some water to cook the dry quinoa. Adjust the heat down to a stew and cover .Cook for 20 minutes or until all the water has evaporated and the quinoa is cushy.

5. Steam or sauté your kale at the same time.

6. In a little pot, whisk together your hot sauce, ghee, and coconut milk. Be sure to set the temperature to medium heat.

7. In a vast skillet, drizzle 1 tbsp. of olive oil and add the diced yellow onion. Cook for 6 minutes or until the onion is translucent.

8. Include the cooked cauliflower and the hot sauce mixture. Combine well to coat all the cauliflower and onion in the sauce.

9. Take a big scoop of quinoa, a bunch of chickpeas, and kale. Include a handful of cauliflower and some diced avocado. Top off the entire bowl with some crisp parsley and dig in!

Zucchini Noodles with Garlic

Total Prep & Cooking Time: 10 Minutes
Yields: 2 Servings

What's in it:

- Zucchini (2 whole)
- EV olive oil (1 tbsp.)
- Garlic powder (1/4 tsp.)
- Garlic salt (1/4 tsp.)
- Pepper to taste

How it's made:

1. Use a spiralizer to make zucchini noodles.

2. Put a skillet on the stove over medium to high heat.

3. Put the zucchini noodles on a cutting board and chop up a few pieces while the skillet is warming up.

4. When the skillet is hot, include EVOO and noodles. Allow them to cook for about 1-2 minutes, then add the seasonings. Cook for an extra 2-3 minutes. The noodles should be tender but slightly firm at the same time.

Curry-Flavored Sweet Potato Tofu

Total Prep & Cooking Time: 25 Minutes
Yields: 2 Servings

What's in it:

- Coconut oil (2 tbsp.)
- Yellow onion (1, finely chopped)
- Ginger garlic paste (1 tbsp.)
- Sweet potato (1 large)
- Green beans (1 cup)
- Yellow bell pepper (1, cut into cubes)
- Red bell pepper (1, cut into cubes)
- Coconut milk + equal quantity water (1 can)
- Tofu (14 oz.; cut and cubed)
- Green chilies (6-7; ground into a chunky paste)
- Curry leaves (1-2 strands)
- Turmeric (2 tsp.)
- Cumin (1/2 tsp.)
- Salt (1 tsp.)

For the Garnish

- Large handful of roasted whole nuts
- Cooked rice (2 cups)

- Green onions, sliced (2-3)
- Chili flakes (pinch)

How it's made:

1. Add oil to a wok pan on medium heat.

2. Add ground green beans and stew. Let it sear until it is delicately sautéed.

3. Include the finely diced onion and ginger garlic paste to the skillet along with the turmeric and cumin.

4. Stir and cook for a couple of minutes until the onion is translucent and caramelized.

5. In the meantime, peel and cut the sweet potato into small cubes. Add the sweet potato to the pan and sauté for a couple of minutes. Mix. You can include a sprinkle of water or more oil if the ingredients stick to the base of the skillet.

6. Include the green beans and bell peppers to the dish and let it sear for 4-5 minutes.

7. Add the coconut milk, water, curry leaves, and tofu. Cook until the sweet potato cubes are soft. This takes around 10-15 minutes. Taste and, if needed, add more flavoring.

8. Serve with some cooked rice, peanuts, green onions, and crushed red chili flakes for that spicy kick.

Fresh Beets with Polenta

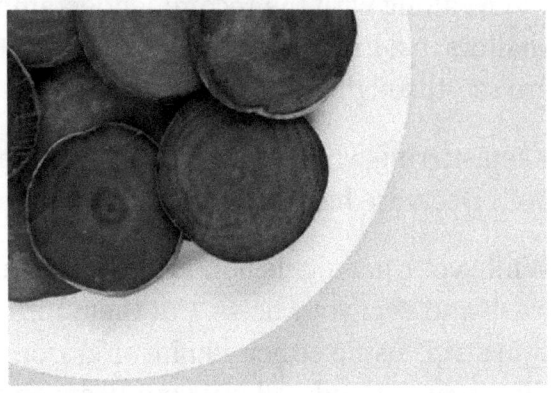

Total Prep & Cooking Time: 25 Minutes
Yields: 4 Servings

What's in it:

1. EV olive oil (3 tbsp.)
2. Shallot (1 large; finely minced)
3. Polenta (2 cups)
4. Water (6 cups)
5. Sea salt and pepper (as desired)
6. Golden beets (2 medium)
7. Olive spray

How it's made:

1. Preset the oven to 350°F and place some parchment paper in the bottom of a baking sheet or flat pan.

2. In a very large skillet on high temperature, add EVOO along with the recommended amount of shallots in a low heat setting; cook until they are see-through.

3. Keep stirring while you bring the polenta to a boil. Decrease heat to a simmer then cover.

4. While your polenta is boiling, go ahead and wash and peel your beets. Cut them into very thin strips using either a knife or grater. Spray the paper with oil and put your beets on it; give them a spray and a dash of the sea salt and pepper.

5. Bake in the oven for 20 minutes; turn it halfway through cooking. You can store the food for up to 5 days if it's in an airtight container and is kept in the fridge.

Shrimp, Soba Noodles, and Sweet Potatoes

Total Prep & Cooking Time: 30 Minutes
Yields: 4-6 Servings

What's in it:

- Sweet potato (1 pound; peeled and cut into 1/2-inch cubes)
- Sea salt (1/8 tsp.)
- Small shrimp (12 oz.)
- Buckwheat soba noodles, 100% (8 oz.)
- Sugar snap peas (8 oz)
- Tahini (1/4 cup)
- Lemon juice (about 3 tbsp.)
- Garlic, minced (2 cloves)
- Crushed red chili flakes (1/4 tsp.)

How it's made:

1. Preset the oven to 425°F. In a baking pan lined with parchment paper, spread the sweet potatoes and sprinkle with salt. Roast for 15 minutes.

2. Remove the pan from the oven, push potatoes to one side, and spread frozen shrimp on the other side. Continue roasting until the shrimp

are just cooked and the potatoes are browned and tender. This takes about 8-10 minutes.

3. Meanwhile, fill a large saucepan halfway with water and stir occasionally to keep the noodles from sticking together; cook just until tender about 6 minutes.

4. Place snap peas in a colander and drain the noodles; rinse in cold water. Toss with the mixture and serve hot.

Spaghetti Squash with Shrimp

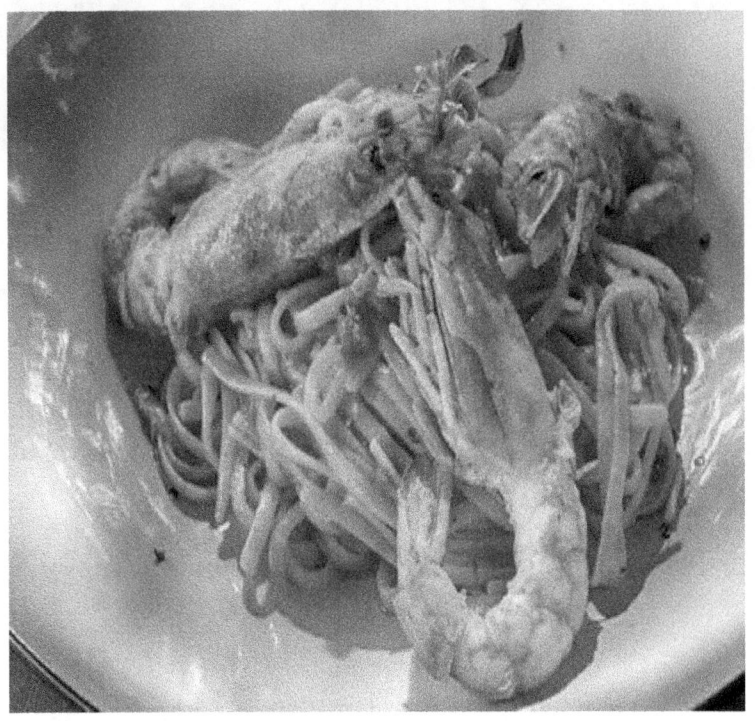

Total Prep & Cooking Time: 1 Hour
Yields: 2 Servings

What's in it:

- Spaghetti squash (1 large)
- Shrimp (1 pound; peeled and deveined)
- Coconut oil (1 tbsp.)
- Salt and pepper

How it's made:

1. Slice the spaghetti squash lengthwise into two pieces. Scoop out the seeds and pulp until it's smooth inside.

2. Place the squash with the cut side up on a steamer or in a pressure cooker. Add 1 cup of water to the bottom and cover. Cook for 5 minutes.

3. When the spaghetti is done cooking, release the valve at the top and let the steam escape. If you don't have a pressure steamer pot, place the spaghetti squash in the oven at 400°F and cook it for about 40 minutes or until cooked through.

4. In the meantime, heat a medium skillet with coconut oil.

5. Wash and pat the shrimp dry, season with salt and pepper, and add to the pan. Cook until the shrimp is opaque on each side, which takes about 3-5 minutes.

6. When the squash has chilled, take a fork and run it in through the pasta, making sure all of the strands are not stuck together. Continue until you get to the outer skin. Arrange in a bowl and put the shrimp on top. Enjoy!

Chicken Burgers with Basil and Zucchini

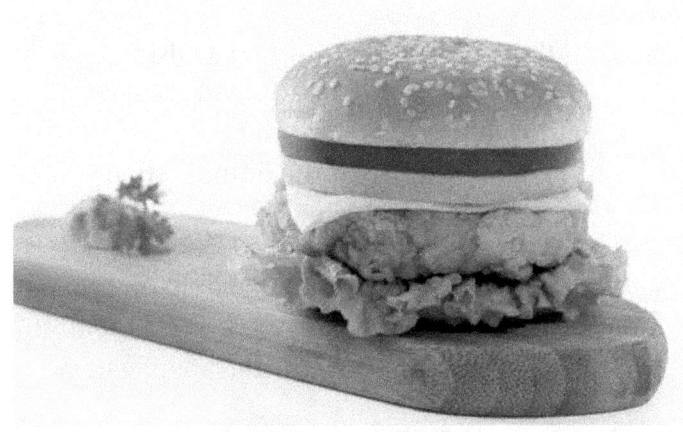

Total Prep & Cooking Time: 20 Minutes
Yields: 4 Servings

What's in it:

- Organic ground chicken (1 pound)
- Zucchini (1 large)
- Sweet onions, diced (1/2 cup)
- Celery, diced (1/2 cup)
- Garlic, minced (2 cloves)
- Fresh basil, chopped (1/4 cup)
- Ghee or avocado oil (2 tbsp.)
- Salt and pepper to taste

How it's made:

1. Place the box grater over a piece of cheesecloth and grate the zucchini.

2. Fold in the corners of the cloth and squeeze out the excess juice into a jar for future use(this is great for smoothies).Salt the zucchini, let the salt bring out more of the liquids, then squeeze it once again into the jar.

3. Add 1 tbsp. of the ghee or avocado oil to a pan over medium heat. Once warm, add the onions and cook 5-10 minutes until translucent.

4. Add the celery and cook for about 3 minutes. Finally, add the garlic and stir for about a minute; remove from heat.

5. In a glass bowl, put the chicken, zucchini, onion-celery-garlic mixture, and basil; thoroughly season with salt and pepper, then form about 4-5 hamburger-sized patties.

6. Add the other tablespoon of ghee or avocado oil to a pan over medium heat. Place each patty in the hot skillet

7. Cook for about 6 minutes per side or until they're completely cooked through. Top with guacamole or your favorite Wholefood condiments.

Shrimp & Pineapple Salad

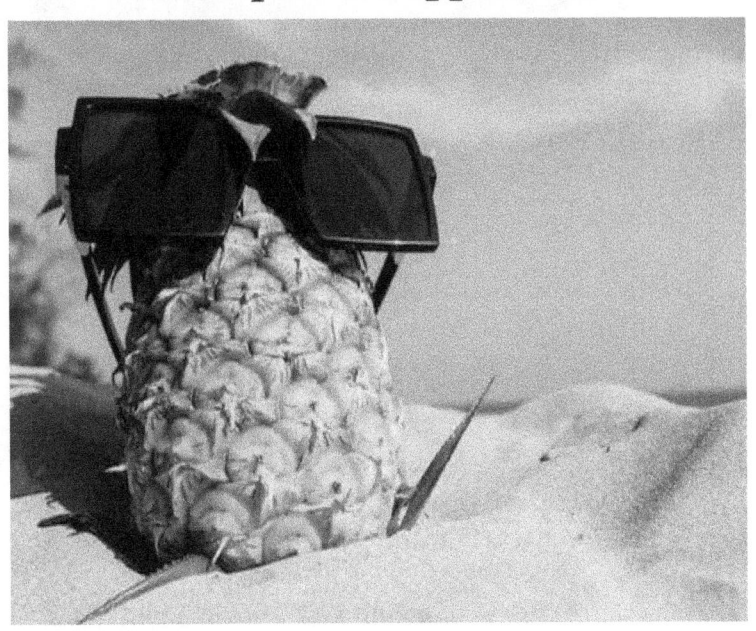

Total Prep & Cooking Time: 15 Minutes
Yields: 4 Servings

What's in it:

- Pineapple (1 large)
- English cucumber, diced (1)
- Jalapeno (½; seeds removed)
- Avocado, diced (1)
- Lime juice (1 lime)
- Sriracha (1/4 tsp.)
- Fresh cilantro, chopped (1/4 cup)
- Cooked shrimp (1 pound)
- Salt and pepper

How it's made:

1. Slice the pineapples down the center. Cut around the perimeter of the inside to score the flesh.

2. Take one-fourth of the insides and use it to create a juice by straining it. Chop the remainder into bite-sized chunks. Combine the cucumber, jalapeno, avocado, lime, shrimp, and the correct quantity of cilantro; add the sriracha to the pineapple and mix it all at once. Season with salt and pepper to taste.

3. The flavors can develop the longer you let it sit; however, the juice will still "cook" the shrimp. It is not advisable to leave it in the fridge for too long. Take a scoop and place the pineapple mixture into the cleaned-out pineapples or a plate and serve.

Chicken Salad with a Kick

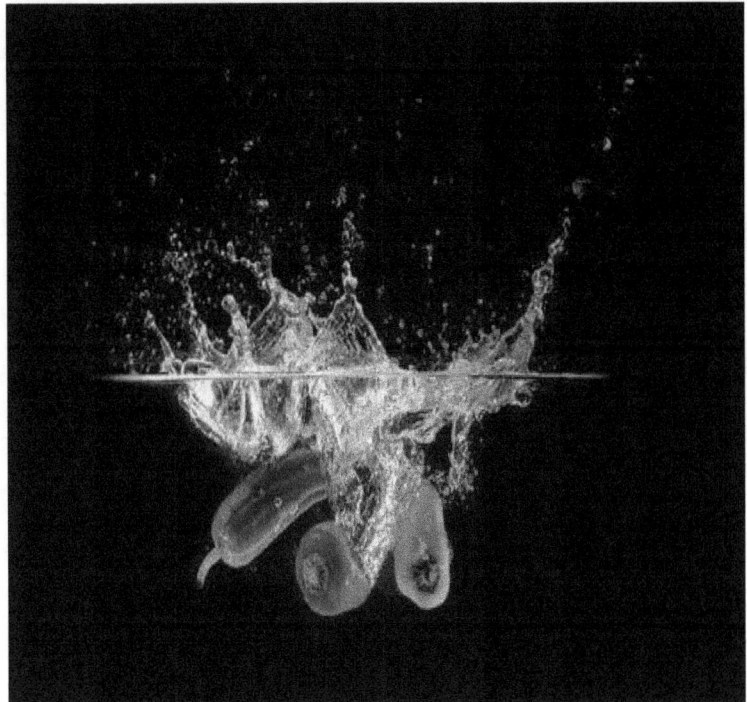

Total Prep & Cooking Time: 10 Minutes
Yields: 4 Servings

What's in it:

- White pepper, ground (1 tsp.)
- Sugar (1 tbsp.)
- Sea salt (½ tsp.)
- White pepper (¼ tsp.)
- Powdered mustard (¼ tsp.)
- Cider vinegar (2 ½ tbsp.)
- Water (3 tbsp.)
- Egg yolk, lightly beaten (1)
- Mayonnaise (2/3 cup)

- Chicken, cubed (5 cups)
- Celery, diced (3 stalks) \
- Red onion, chopped (½)
- Preferred whole food dressing (2/3 cup)
- Sour cream (1/2 cup)
- Sea salt (2 tsp.)

How it's made:

Make the Dressing:

1. Grab a bowl and whisk together the sugar, flour, salt and pepper, and mustard; put it aside on the counter.
2. In a saucepan, be sure to bring the vinegar and water to a high boil. Using extreme caution, add the boiled mixture to the egg yolk, stir often until it's warm all the way through. If any egg happens to get hard, simply pick it out and throw it away.
3. Slowly stir in all of the wet ingredients with the dry ingredients, mixing constantly until everything is well-incorporated.
4. Reduce heat to the low setting and pour the mixture back into the pan. Be sure to stir it often and then heat the mixture until it is as thick as you want it. Do not bring it to a complete boil. Take off of the heat and put it in a bowl to let it cool off. Mix it after cooling.

Make the Chicken Salad:

1. Put celery and red onion in food processor and pulse; you can also simply chop it by hand. Return it to the final bowl.

2. Add chicken to the serving bowl. Combine the cooked chicken, celery, diced red onion, and dressing. Feel free to add more salt and pepper to your preference.

Barley Soup

Total Prep & Cooking Time: 8 Hours and 10 Minutes
Yields: 11 Servings

What's in it:

- Yellow onion, chopped (1)
- Carrots (2; cut into 1/2-inch circles)
- Celery, chopped (2 stalks)
- Sweet potato (1; cut into 1/4-inch pieces)
- Garlic , minced (4 cloves)
- Frozen green beans (1 1/2 cups)
- Pearl barley (3/4 cup)
- Paprika (1 tsp.)
- Dried oregano (1 tsp.)
- Dried thyme (3/4 tsp.)
- Salt (1/2 tsp.)
- Ground pepper (1/2 tsp.)
- Petite diced tomatoes (1 14-oz. can)
- Vegetable broth (6 cups; low-sodium)
- Water (2 cups)
- Flat-leaf parsley, minced (1/4 cup)

How it's made:

1. Combine all the ingredients in a Crockpot, leaving out the parsley for garnishing when it's finished cooking.
2. Cook on a low heat setting until the barley is tender when forked, which typically takes 8 hours.

3. Add the parsley on top. Serve.

Mushroom and Spinach Frittata

Total Prep & Cooking Time: 10 Minutes
Yields: 8 Servings

What's in it:

- Ghee butter (2 tbsp.)
- Fresh baby spinach (3 cups)
- Fresh sliced mushrooms (1 cup)
- Eggs (8 large)
- Soy milk (¼ cup)
- Vegan cheese or any alternative to cheese (½ cup; crumbles)
- Salt and pepper to taste

How it's made:

1. Start by heating the oven broiler to high. In a skillet on top of the stove, melt the butter on medium heat. Next, add your mushrooms and cook them approximately 2 minutes, stirring often until the mushrooms are soft.
2. Add the spinach and cook for another 1 minute until the spinach has wilted. Mix together the eggs and milk in a bowl and season to your liking.
3. Put the eggs in the skillet and cook for 3-4 minutes, stirring every minute or so. Once the eggs begin to set but are still slightly runny on top, sprinkle on the cheese.
4. Put the skillet under the broiler; cook for 1-2 minutes until the eggs are set and the cheese begins to melt.

5. Cut the frittata and serve. Enjoy!

Dessert Recipes

Try these delicious recipes and discover that even a whole food diet has room for dessert!

Cashew and Chocolate Cupcakes

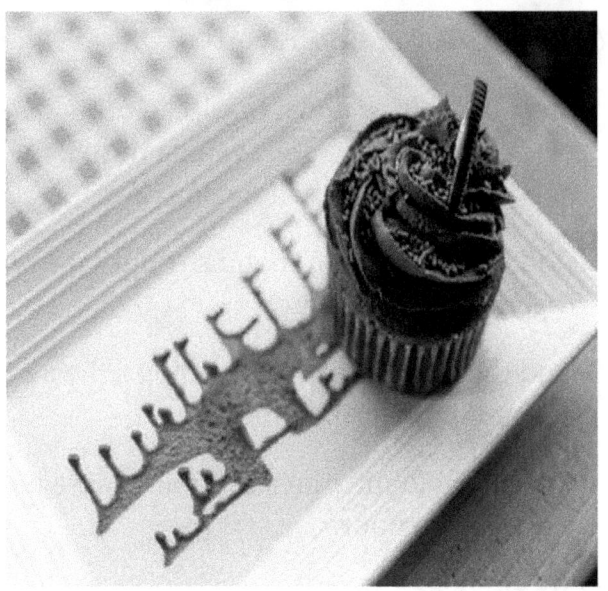

Total Prep & Cooking Time: 4 Hours
Yields: 9 Servings

What's in it:

- Cacao powder (1 cup)
- Cacao butter, melted (1 cup)
- Agave nectar (1/3 cup)
- Vanilla bean powder (1 tbsp.)
- Cashews (1 cup; soaked for 4 hours)
- Coconut oil (½ cup)
- Filtered water (½ cup)
- Himalayan salt to taste

How it's made:

To Make the Chocolate Base:

1. Start by melting down the cacao butter. Next, place the cacao powder, vanilla bean powder, and cashew cream in a mixing bowl.

2. Add the melted butter and stir until it's mixed together with no lumps.

3. Add the chocolate mixture using a measuring cup and pour into a cupcake pan.

4. Put the mold into the freezer and leave it for at least half an hour.

To Make the Cashew Cream:

1. Clean and wash the cashews extremely well; put everything in the blender until it is all smooth.

2. Remove the cupcake mold from the freezer and add the cashew cream on top of each cupcake. Place them back in the freezer overnight.

3. After you remove them from the freezer, allow to set for at least half an hour before serving.

Coconut and Berry Cake

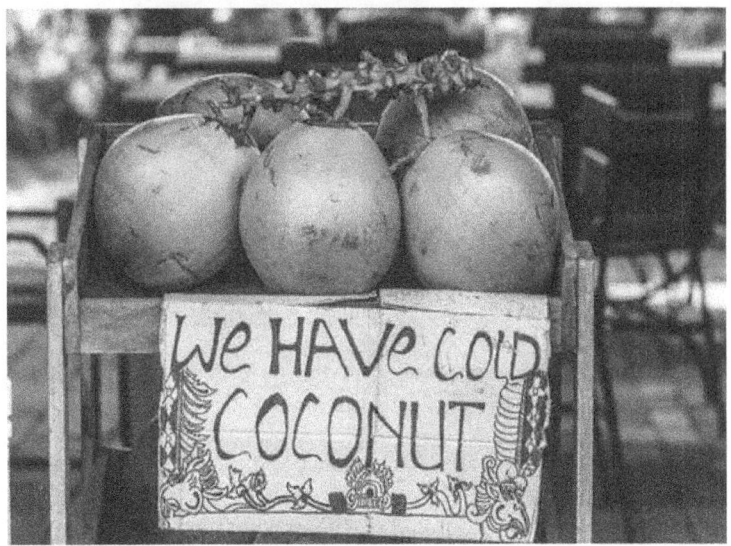

Total Prep & Cooking Time: 35 Minutes
Yields: 16 Servings

What's in it:

For the Dough:

- Gluten-free flour of choice (4 cups)
- Dates (10; chopped)
- Coconut oil (1/2 cup)
- Cacao (1 cup)
- Plant-based milk (2 cups)
- Water (1 cup)
- Aluminum-free baking powder (2 tbsp.)
- Baking soda (2 tsp.)
- Dash of salt
- Organic vanilla (1 tbsp.)

Forthe Coconut Cream:

- Coconut cream (3.5 oz.)
- Coconut yogurt (3.5 oz.)
- Vanilla agar -optional (1 tbsp.)

Forthe Topping:

- Berries (strawberries, raspberries, blueberries, etc.)
- Vegan white chocolate for sprinkling
- Coconut flakes

How it's made:

1. First, chop the dates. Add all the dry ingredients in a bowl and mix well.
2. Next, add the milk and water. Be careful that the dough does not become thin. Lastly, add in the chopped dates.
3. Set the oven to 390°F. Line a round spring form pan either with parchment paper or with coconut oil. Pour the dough and distribute evenly. Bake for about 30 minutes and let it cool off.
4. Slowly heat the coconut cream to thin it out.
5. Next, mix all the ingredients together. Before you serve this dish, add the berries on top. If you wish, you can melt the white chocolate and top the cake with it as well as add some coconut flakes.

Salted Caramel Bites

Total Prep & Cooking Time: 20 Minutes
Yields: 10 Servings

What's in it:

- Coconut oil (1/3 cup)
- Tahini (1/2 cup; raw)
- Dates (1 cup, pitted)
- Sea salt (1/4 tsp.)

How it's made:

1. Start by pre-soaking the dates in hot water for about 10 minutes.

2. As they are pre-soaking, proceed to combine the melted coconut oil and tahini together in a bowl.

3. Take only 1 tbsp. of the mixture and place it into muffin tins; then, place them in the freezer to form. This process should only take 5-10 minutes.

4. After it has formed, blend the dates along with the sea salt until they are completely smooth and creamy.

5. Divide the remaining date mixture into the rest of the muffin pan and add the remaining tahini mixture over the top.

6. Place the pan back into the freezer until they're formed; this usually takes about 20-30 minutes. Serve and enjoy!

Ice Cream

Total Prep & Cooking Time: 10 Minutes
Yields: 4 Servings

What's in it:

1. Medium ripe bananas (8, peeled)

How it's made:

1. Chop your bananas into 1-inch cubes. Put them on a plate in a single layer and freeze until solid; it would take a minimum of 2 hours.

2. Place the frozen banana items in a food processor and puree until creamy(2-3 minutes), scraping the edges of the processor to get all of it out.

3. This frozen dessert is often served cold and can have a texture similar to soft serve.Let the frozen dessert soften at least ten minutes before serving.

Chocolate Cupcakes

Total Prep & Cooking Time: 40 Minutes
Yields: 6 Servings

What's in it:

- Dates (1 cup; deseeded)
- Oat flour (1 cup)
- Water (1 cup)
- Leavening (1 tbsp.)
- Plant-based milk (1/4 cup)
- Cacao tree powder (1/4 cup)

Chocolate Icing:

- Dates (1 cup; deseeded)
- Plant-based milk (2/3 cup)
- Cacao powder (2 tbsp)

Coconut Topping Icing:

- Coconut milk (1 cup; chilled)

How it's made:

Chocolate Icing:

1. Combine all of the frosting ingredients in a mixer and blend on high until it's smooth lump-free. Chill in the fridge for a minimum of 2 hours.

Coconut Icing:

1. Whip until smooth.

Cupcakes:

2. Heat up the oven to 350°F.

3. Blend the dates and water until the mixture is sleek. A high-speed mixer works best.

4. Add the oat flour, leavening, chocolate, and non-dairy milk. Mix until well-combined.

5. Spoon the batter into six lined or oiled quick bread tins. Fill them three-quarters of the way. Bake at 350°F for about 25 minutes.

6. Remove from the pan and allow them to cool. Apply the icing. Serve and enjoy!

Whole Food Bars and Balls

Total Prep & Cooking Time: 15 Minutes
Yields: 30 Servings

What's in it:

- Protein-free oatmeal (2 cups)
- Pumpkin seeds (½ cup)
- Hemp seeds (one cup)
- Cacao nibs (½ cup)
- Pecans (1 cup)
- Goji berries (½ cup)
- Dates (1 cup)
- Vanilla powder (1 tsp.)
- Sea salt (pinch)
- Water (½ to ¾ cup)

How it's made:

1. Place oats, pumpkin seeds, hemp seeds, cacao nibs, and pecans in an adequate-sized bowl.

2. Place goji berries in a smaller container and fill with heated water. Soak for 5 minutes or until they soften a bit.

3. Once slightly soft, drain the water and place the berries into the bowl with the remainder of the ingredients.

4. Place dates, flavoring, salt, and water in a blender or high-speed processor. Combine until the mixture is partly smooth and partly chunky.

5. Combine the mixture with the remainder of the ingredients into a bowl. Mix until you get a dough-like consistency.

6. Place the mixture into a square baking dish lined with parchment and press firmly.

7. Roll the mixture into balls and coat with coconut flakes.

Chocolate Chip and Caramel Cookies with No Flour

Total Prep & Cooking Time: 20 Minutes
Yields: 8 Servings

What's in it:

- Cashew butter (1 cup)
- Dates, pitted (5; soak for 5 minutes)
- Water (2 tbsp.)
- Ground vanilla beans (1 tsp.)
- Sea salt (1/4 tsp.)
- Leavening (1/4 tsp.)
- Sugar-free chocolate chips (1/4 cup)

How it's made:

1. Preheat your stove or oven to 350°F. Strain the dates.

2. In a mixer, blend the dates, sea salt, and water until a caramel-like texture is achieved.

3. In a separate bowl, combine the cashew butter, vanilla, and leavening. Add the caramel to the cashew butter mixture and pulse a couple of times.

4. Lastly, add the chocolate chips and pulse a couple of times. Put the dough on a cookie

sheet or lined baking pan and bake for 10 minutes. Do not take them off the sheet until they have fully cooled off.

5. You may store the cookies in a sealed container and refrigerate for up to2 weeks.

Orange Chocolate Pudding –Post-30-Day Challenge Recipe

Total Prep & Cooking Time: 20 Minutes
Yields: 2 Servings

What's in it:

- Vanilla powder (½ tsp.)
- Avocado (1)
- Dates (1 cup)
- Dark/unsweetened chocolate(1/3 cup)
- Orange zest (1 tsp.)
- Orange juice(1/2 cup)
- Sea salt (1/8 tsp.)

How it's made:

1. In a food processor, puree all the ingredients until the mixture is completely smooth with no lumps. Repeatedly pause the processor to scrape down the sides. Note that this pudding is incredibly thick. If you wish to thin it, you can add water or coconut milk until it's at the desired consistency.

2. Serve or store in the fridge.

Chia Seed and Mango Pudding

Total Prep & Cooking Time: 1 hour
Yields: 4 Servings

What's in it:

- Coconut milk (2 cups)
- Chia seeds (1/2 cup)
- Vanilla powder (1 tsp.)
- Cardamom (1/4 tsp.)
- Mango (2 medium)
- Coconut nectar (3 tbsp.)

How it's made:

1. In a sealable container, add the milk, chia seeds, vanilla powder, cardamom, and cinnamon. Whisk all the ingredients together and put it in the fridge overnight.

2. When the pudding has set, slice the mango and place in a blender. Add a tablespoon of coconut milk and blend until it reaches a smooth creamy texture.

3. In your favorite serving dishes, place layers of the pudding and the mango cream until you reach the top of the dish. Leave a little room on top for a sprinkle of chia seeds. Serve cold and enjoy!

Banana Bread Cookies —Post-30-Day Challenge Recipe

Total Prep & Cooking Time: 25 Minutes
Yields: 18 Servings

What's in it:

- Ripe bananas (2)
- Ghee butter (½ cup)
- Maple or agave syrup (2 tbsp.)
- Oats (2 cups)
- Chia seeds (1 tbsp.)
- Cinnamon (1 tsp.)
- Sea salt (¼ tsp.)
- Nutmeg (dash)
- Mini chocolate chips (¼ cup)

How it's made:

1. Preheat your oven to 350°F.

2. Mash the bananas in a large bowl. Add the butter and syrup and blend well.

3. Stir in the oats, chia seeds, cinnamon, and nutmeg; blend until you have a thick batter. Fold in the chocolate chips.

4. Scoop out chunks (about 2 tbsp. per ball). Wet your hands and then roll them around to form balls. They will flatten into cookie form while baking.

5. Bake for 14-15 minutes. Remove them from the oven and let them cool for at least 10 minutes before serving.

Buckwheat Granola Bars with Peanut Butter

Total Prep & Cooking Time: 30 Minutes
Yields: 15-16 Servings

What's in it:

- Puffed buckwheat (1½ cup)
- Peanut butter (⅓ cup)
- Maple or agave syrup (¼ cup +2 tbsp.)
- Dark chocolate chips (⅓ cup)
- Cinnamon (1 tsp.)
- Cocoa (1 tsp.)
- Ginger (½ tsp.)
- Raisins
- Chia seeds or flax seeds

How it's made:

1. Line a glass baking pan with parchment paper.

2. Heat a large pan over medium heat and pour the syrup and butter.

3. Reduce heat to low and stir with a wooden spoon.

4. When the syrup and butter are melted, turn off the fire and add the puffed buckwheat's.

5. Stir well to mix until the buckwheat's are well-coated. Place the pot back on the fire for 30 seconds if necessary.

6. Transfer the mixture to a baking pan and cover it with another sheet of parchment paper .Using a spatula, spread the ingredients well to form a packed layer. It's important that it's packed well or the bars will crumble once cut.

7. Place in the fridge to cool for 5 minutes, then take the whole bar mixture out of the baking pan.

8. If you're making energy bars, drizzle glaze over the mixture with a teaspoon. Let it cool and proceed to cut them in to your preferred serving shape and size.

For the Chocolate Glaze:

1. Microwave the chocolate in a glass dish for 30 seconds. Whisk and heat until dissolved.

2. Dip the cookie-like bars into the dissolved chocolate and let cool.

Rainbow Fruit with Black Rice

Total Prep & Cooking Time: 2 Hours 5 Minutes
Yields: 1 Serving

What's in it:

- Coconut milk (⅓ cup)
- Chia seeds (1 tbsp.)
- Matcha powder (1 tsp.)
- Cooked black sticky rice (⅓ cup)
- Nectarine, chopped (1)
- Pomegranate (¼; arils only)
- Fruit (1/2 cup; for garnish)

How it's made:

1. At least two hours beforehand, mix chia seeds, coconut milk, and matcha powder in a large bowl. Set aside in the fridge.

2. Prepare the fruit.

3. Spoon half the black sticky rice in a glass or jar. Pour some coconut milk over the rice, if desired.

4. Continue to layer your glass or jar with pomegranate arils, nectarine, the remaining black rice, and the matcha chia pudding.

5. Garnish with more fruit or as desired.

Easy Cheesecake

Total Prep & Cooking Time: 1 Hour and 10 Minutes
Yields: 4 Servings

What's in it:

- Cashews (1½ cups)
- Dates (8; soft, pitted)
- Cashew butter (2 tbsp.)

Filling:
Raw cashews (1 cup; pre-soaked and strained)
Vanilla coconut yogurt (1 cup)
Agave (6 tbsp.)
Lemon juice (1)
Psyllium husk (1 tbsp.)
Pure vanilla extract (1 tsp.)
Salt (1 tsp.)
Ground vanilla bean, raw (1 tsp.)

How it's made:

Start by preheating the oven to 350°F. Lightly oil a 6-inchspringform pan (base and sides) and set aside.
Add all the dry ingredients in a food processor and run until the mixture is a fine sticky crumble. Transfer into the oiled pan; press down with your hands to form a crust on the bottom and sides of the pan.
Set aside while you blend all of the filling ingredients together.
Bake for 40-45 minutes until it is sweet-smelling and golden. Leave to cool for 10 minutes. Add the filling. Slice and serve.

Cauliflower Chocolate Pudding

Total Prep & Cooking Time: 20 Minutes
Yields: 2 Servings

What's in it:

- Cauliflower florets (3 cups)
- Non-dairy milk (2 cups)
- Cacao powder (1/3 cup)
- Dates (10; pitted)
- Vanilla bean powder (1/2 tsp.)

How it's made:

1. Steam the cauliflower until it is extremely soft and tender.

2. Blend all the ingredients in your food processor until it has a smooth, creamy texture.

3. You can choose to chill it in the fridge or eat it immediately. This will keep in a covered container for up to 24 hours in the fridge.

Snack Recipes

Try these delicious snacks that are not only made of real whole foods but are also as healthy as they are tasty!

No-Bake Energy Balls

Total Prep & Cooking Time: 20 Minutes
Yields: 12 Servings

What's in it:

- Ghee (½ cup)
- Hemp hearts (½ cup)
- Sugarless coconut flakes (3/4 cup)
- Vanilla (1 tsp.)
- Pie spice (1 tbsp.)
- Dates (10; large)
- Dried raisins (¾ cup)

How it's made:

1. In a high-speed mixer or food processor, mix the almond butter, hemp hearts, half a cup of coconut flakes, vanilla, and pie spice until they're well-combined. Fold dates into the batter.

2. Scoop the dough with a small ice cream scoop into tablespoon-sized balls. Roll the balls until they're firm and well-packed, then sprinkle with the rest of the coconut.

3. Eat right away or store in a fridge until you're ready to eat. This can be kept for up to 2 weeks.

Banana Sushi

Total Prep & Cooking Time: 10 Minutes
Yields: 1 Servings

What's in it:

- Banana (1)
- Nut butter paste (1 tbsp.)
- Optional toppings: chia seeds, coconut

How it's made:

1. Peel the banana and then layer with1 tbsp. of nut butter paste.

2. Sprinkle with optional toppings and press them gently into the nut butter to make sure they'll stick.

3. Using a sharp knife, slice the banana much like how you would slice sushi.

4. Serve cold or as is. Enjoy this no-cook, guilt-free snack!

Fruit Skewers

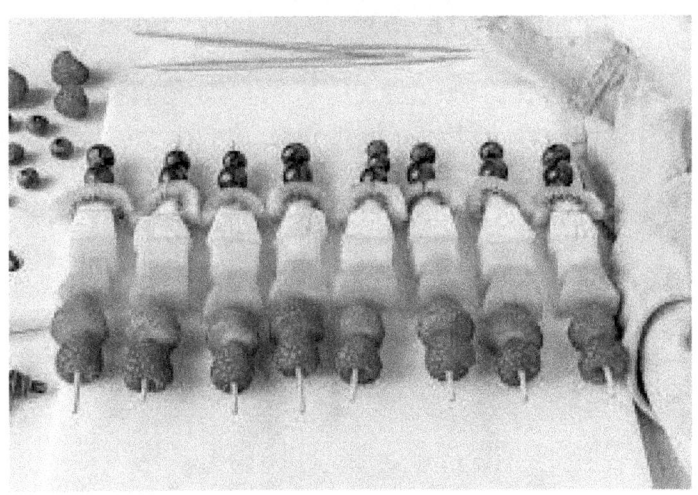

Total Prep & Cooking Time: 10 Minutes
Yields: 8 Skewers

What's in it:

- Pineapple (1/2; diced and cubed)
- Nectarines (3-4; diced and cubed)
- Plums (3-4; diced and cubed)
- Peaches (3-4; diced and cubed)
- Pears (3-4; diced and cubed)
- Apricots (3-4; diced and cubed)
- Strawberries (10-15; tops and bottoms cut off)
- Oranges (3 large; cut and segmented)

How it's made:

1. Chop the fruits into bite-sized pieces then alternate them on skewers/barbeque sticks.

2. You can place them in baggies and freeze for later or put them in containers for snacks you can grab on the go.

Cucumber Boats with Hummus

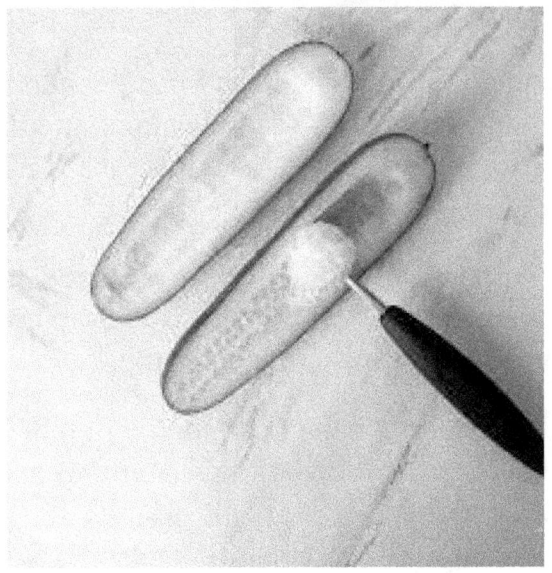

Total Prep & Cooking Time: 15 Minutes
Yields: 24 Servings

What's in it:

- Garbanzo beans (32 oz.)
- EV olive oil (2 tbsp.)
- Juice (your choice; 3 tbsp.)
- Paprika (2 tsp.)
- Cayenne pepper (2 tsp.)
- Sea salt (1 tsp.)
- Cucumbers (12; baby sized)

How it's made:

1. You'll want to grab at least one pastry bag or a Ziploc bag.

2. Put all the ingredients in a blender and mix until you no longer see any lumps and the texture is creamy. Add additional salt if you prefer.

3. Wash and slice the cucumbers lengthwise. Scoop out half of the flesh or you can leave it as is and place the hummus on top.

4. Put a quarter cup of hummus within the bag. Fill the cucumbers with the hummus and use a little sprinkle of paprika if desired.

5. You can chill the cucumbers before serving or eat immediately!

Fresh Fruit Snacks

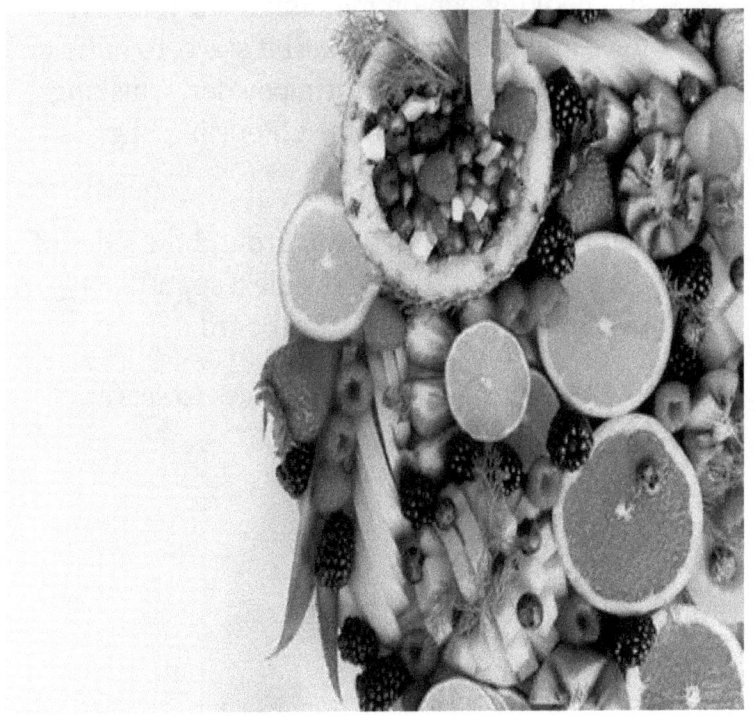

Total Prep & Cooking Time: 30 Minutes
Yields: 8 Servings

What's in it:

- Pureed fruit (1 1/2 cups)
- Unflavored gelatin powder (1/4 cup)
- Honey (2 tbsp.)
- Fruit crush (3 tbsp.)

How it's made:

1. Puree fruit in a blender. Pour it into a medium-size cooking pan on medium heat. Whisk in juice and honey. Heat until it starts to bubble and slowly add the gelatin powder, whisking frequently until combined. Pour into a glass baking dish.

2. After the mixture sets, cut around the sides of the pan with a knife and slide a spatula beneath; place on a cutting board.

3. Cut the fruit into bite-size pieces to serve.

Conclusion

Thank you for making it to the end of *The 30-Day Whole Food Challenge: A Guide to a "Whole" New You*. We hope it was informative and able to provide you with all the tools you need to achieve your healthy eating goals, weight loss goals, or simply your goal to live a better life.

The next step is to begin the preparation for your lifestyle change. While this book is mostly about food, that is not all that the challenge is about. Try to get enough sleep each night and find creative ways to say no to your junk cravings and avoid your guilty pleasures. Begin to meditate if you don't already and focus on being less stressed about your food decisions. Slowly, you will see a boost in your confidence and self-assurance.

Take the meal plan that we provided and plan your meals for 30 days using the recipes in the book. You could also do some research and come up with recipes of your own. As mentioned before, remove or give away all the food items you should not have in your home. If you are the only one in your family doing the challenge, be sure to separate your food from the rest of the family's so you won't be tempted to cheat the challenge and so they won't accidentally eat what you have prepared for yourself. Not that it would be a bad thing if they did, but if you are portioning out food for the week, you don't want to be forced to cheat because you are short on planned snacks and meals. Remember, every time you cheat, you have to go back to square one.

Begin a journal and start documenting how you feel 24 hours after consuming whichever food a day before. This will not only help you develop a healthy relationship with the food that makes you feel certain ways, it would also help you create a more efficient way of meal planning. For example, if you have a big exam coming up or a huge presentation to give at work and you know that eating broccoli makes you gassy, then you would know it's not the best choice for that day.

Get your kitchen in order with all the utensils, spices, and kitchen tools that we identified in this book. Do your own research and find tools that you want to use in your new challenge that will help you be successful at staying committed. Ease of access and prepping is a great motivator for sticking with your challenge and staying healthy.

Start with the 7-day kick-start meal plan we provided and, most importantly, have fun on your new journey! This is not going to be easy, but it should be rewarding and fun!

Finally, if you found this book useful in any way, a review on Amazon is always appreciated!

I hope you enjoyed this book! Please be kind enough to leave a review if this book helped you in any way possible, and I hope you succeed at the challenge, all the best!

www.ingramcontent.com/pod-product-compliance
Lightning Source LLC
Chambersburg PA
CBHW051542020426
42333CB00016B/2049